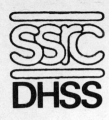

Studies in Deprivation and Disadvantage 5

Mothers and Daughters

A Three-generational Study of Health Attitudes and Behaviour

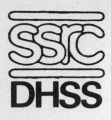

Studies in Deprivation and Disadvantage

Despite substantial economic advances and improved welfare services in Britain since the Second World War, there has been a conspicuous persistence of deprivation and maladjustment. In June 1972 Sir Keith Joseph, then Secretary of State for Social Services, drew attention to this. In particular it seemed to him that social problems tended to recur in successive generations of the same families – to form a 'cycle of deprivation'. Subsequently the Department of Health and Social Security, through the Social Science Research Council, made available a sum of money for a programme of research into the whole problem.

Academics and practitioners from a wide range of disciplines and professional backgrounds were invited to investigate many aspects of deprivation and the process of transmission. Their findings are now becoming available and many of the empirical studies, together with literature reviews and the final summary report on deprivation and social policy, are being published in this series of *Studies in Deprivation and Disadvantage*.

1 Cycles of Disadvantage: A Review of Research
Michael Rutter and Nicola Madge

2 A Cycle of Deprivation? A Case Study of Four Families
Frank Coffield, Philip Robinson and Jacquie Sarsby

3 The Health of the Children: A Review of Research on the Place of Health in Cycles of Disadvantage
Mildred Blaxter

4 Disadvantage and Education
Jo Mortimore and Tessa Blackstone

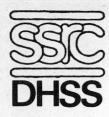

Studies in Deprivation and Disadvantage 5

Mothers and Daughters

A Three-generational Study of Health Attitudes and Behaviour

*Mildred Blaxter and Elizabeth Paterson
with the assistance of Sheila Murray*

Heinemann Educational Books · London

Published by Heinemann Educational Books Ltd
22 Bedford Square, London WC1B 3HH
LONDON EDINBURGH MELBOURNE AUCKLAND
HONG KONG SINGAPORE KUALA LUMPUR NEW DELHI
IBADAN NAIROBI JOHANNESBURG
EXETER [NH] KINGSTON PORT OF SPAIN

First published 1982

British Library Cataloguing in Publication Data

Blaxter, Mildred
   Mothers and daughters: a three generational study of health attitudes and
   behaviour.
   —(SSRC/DHSS studies in deprivation and disadvantage;5)
   1. Health
   I. Title II. Paterson, Elizabeth
   III. Series
   613   RA418

   ISBN 0-435-82055-9

Phototypesetting by Georgia Origination, Liverpool
and printed and bound in Great Britain by
Biddles Ltd, Guildford, Surrey

Contents

Acknowledgements

The research project on which this volume is based was supported by the Joint Working Party on Transmitted Deprivation of the Department of Health and Social Security and the Social Science Research Council.

We are grateful to the following for help or critical advice: Professor Raymond Illsley, Institute of Medical Sociology; Dr Barbara Thompson, Institute of Medical Sociology; Professor I. MacGillivray, Department of Obstetrics and Gynaecology, Aberdeen University; Miss Jack, Divisional Nursing Officer, Community Health Division, Grampian Health Board; Dr C. M. T. Robb, Specialist in Community Medicine, Grampian Health Board; Professor A. G. M. Campbell, Department of Child Health, Aberdeen University. Our thanks are due also to all the health visitors who agreed to be interviewed. Above all, we are grateful to all the families who were studied, for their patience and co-operation.

List of Tables

1 Health and the 'Cycle of Deprivation'

In the context of a freely available National Health Service, how is it that successive generations of families in poor circumstances continue to suffer deprivation in health? This question is the starting point for the study described in this volume.

There is a great deal of evidence that those people who suffer social disadvantage of various sorts are likely to experience more illness (especially chronic illness) than those in more fortunate circumstances.[1] Obviously, it is the children who are particularly relevant to any hypothesised 'cycle of disadvantage'. And despite the very real general improvements in child health in Britain, there is known still to be a relative disparity between social groups at birth, and a health deficit among poorer families in childhood. The effects of this may persist to adult life[2] and may have repercussions on the health of the next generation. Health problems are known to be particularly acute among groups who suffer multiple deprivations.[3]

There are certain obvious explanations. Heredity must have a part to play, as must the physical environment. But though the relationship between social disadvantage and health is well established, the nature of the association and the role played by various social, economic and cultural factors is not wholly understood. It is often suggested that aspects of behaviour are involved, since 'those who most need services tend to use them least',[4] and it is in the areas of preventive medicine and health maintenance that there is most concern.

This study began with no assumptions about the existence or nature of any more general 'cycle of disadvantage'. Its objective was to examine, in an exploratory and intensive way rather than at the level of large-scale statistics, the health and health care of children as one possible mechanism in the perpetuation of disadvantage through generations.

Models of Explanation
There is a long research tradition in the sociology of health and

poverty, principally deriving from the United States, which seeks to examine the relationship between attitudes to health and health 'deprivation'. In early work, social maladjustment—of which patterns of health-related behaviour could be a part—was viewed primarily as a function of personality. In the past, the notion of hereditary defect was stressed, giving way more recently to an emphasis on the results of psychosocial deprivation. The work of social anthropologists has been influential in turning attention to what was held to be a well-defined 'culture of poverty', characterised by marginality, a low level of social organisation, helplessness, dependence, and a feeling of inferiority.[5] Apathy and fatalism, it was thought, might explain the underuse by the poor in the United States of medical services, and the low value which appeared to be placed on the maintenance of health. Preventive health behaviour, in particular, requires an orientation towards the future which may be incompatible with fatalism.[6]

This subculture, it was suggested, was alienated from the values of modern medicine. Medical professionals and their middle-class patients shared a rational or scientific approach to health and to the postponement of immediate gratification, but these were foreign to the subculture of poverty.[7] And, essentially, this subculture was self-perpetuating:

> The culture of poverty may originally be based on a history of economic deprivation, but it seems to be a culture exhibiting its own rationale, and structure, and reflecting a way of life that is transmitted to new generations.[8]

In more recent years, this model of a continuing subculture has been severly criticised[9] and has given way to one which emphasises rather the conditions under which health care is given, stressing the practical barriers which may face poorer families. Much attention has been paid to the relationship of various 'predisposing' and 'enabling' factors which may influence health behaviour.[10] This mode of explanation alters the focus of inquiry from the individual patient to the manner of service-delivery, and its possible mismatch with the values of particular groups of clients.[11]

In Britain, in a different society and with a very different system of health care, there has been little work at an equivalent theoretical level, and the relevance of these models has rarely been tested. Evidence about the differential use among social groups of services for the cure of illness is equivocal, though there is certainly long-standing concern that aspects of preventive care (such as antenatal services, or the immunisation of children) are neglected among poorer families.[12] The suggestion is frequently met with among service-providers that it *is* possible to identify families whose health care is inefficient, and whose attitudes to health are passed down from one generation to another.

Echoes of the 'culture of poverty' and of the 'systems barriers' models of explanation for this poor health care may be found in the British literature or in policy statements: it was concluded in a report of the National Child Development Survey, for instance, that

> the answer must surely be that either the statutory services are not in general seen as being relevant to their children's welfare—or else there are barriers, physical and psychological, to their attending[13]

and the Court Report on services for child health commented:

> An effective health service and especially an effective child health service must be knowledgeable about the social and economic circumstances of those it serves and have developed a philosophy of how its expertise and facilities can best be made available to those in need of them.[14]

Aim of the Study

These questions are considered in this study in the particular context of continuity and change within families. The hypothesis with which it began was that perceptions of health experiences might, in poor socioeconomic circumstances, create attitudes of apathy towards health care and conflict with health professionals, and that these attitudes might be transmitted through generations, especially among the female members of the family. The aim was therefore to obtain from an older generation of women information about their past and present perceptions of the structure and functions of health services. These would then be compared with the attitudes of their daughters, young women with children of their own, to see to what extent values and beliefs appeared to be transmitted or to recur throughout generations.

It is, however, the practical consequences of the relationship between attitudinal and behavioural variables which are of the greatest importance, in terms of the health care of the children of the next generation. Therefore it was also proposed to document the health-care behaviour of the mothers in detail over a longitudinal period, in order to examine this relationship. Obviously changes in the structures of service available, and changes in the social environment of the two generations, were factors which had to be taken into consideration. Inevitably, we are dealing with a changing society. However, the effect of social change was minimised by excluding upwardly mobile families and confining the study to daughters who were, like their mothers, in the lowest social classes.

In order to attempt to offer explanations for the health behaviour of these families, it was necessary to try to understand it within their own frame of reference. A further objective of the study was therefore to document the group's social approach to health and illness and their informal body of knowledge, knowledge which, as Fabrega has noted,

> serves as the lay basis of orientation and action towards illness . . . and includes names of illnesses, lay beliefs about causation, standard remedies and routines for home treatment, and a body of rules and expectations which serve to pattern the behaviour of lay persons who are ill and those who come into contact with them.[15]

How this knowledge is learnt is obviously a relevant topic. The study could not hope to explore every aspect of this, but did hope to examine the extent to which health attitudes, knowledge and beliefs are passed from one generation to another. Although there are few studies which have dealt directly with health learning, it is generally believed that patterns of health-service utilisation are acquired within a family setting.[16] There is some agreement on the central role of the mother in the transmission of attitudes,[17] and on the continuing importance of the mother–adult daughter relationship.[18] It has been found, however, that a mother's attitudes are rather poor predictors of attitudes in children,[19] and Litman's study of three-generation families in a midwestern metropolitan area of America suggested that it was generational differences which were most salient.[20] Continuity in attitudes and/or in behaviour might or might not be evident in the group being studied here, and if it were, there might of course be several alternative mechanisms of explanation.

In summary, the following questions are the ones which were being addressed: Is there evidence that the children of these families are indeed 'health deprived', in the sense that their health care is poor and the service-use of the families is troubled? Is this deprivation related to the attitudes to health of the young mothers and their perception of the organisation and function of health services? Are the attitudes of the young mothers, in turn, similar to those of *their* mothers: does it appear that intergenerational continuity exists which has a familial element, and is the result of beliefs and experiences overtly shared between the generations? Or does it seem that any apparent continuity is due rather to continuity in the socioeconomic or cultural environment?

As the following chapters will show, our conclusion is that the original hypothesis about the transmission of health deprivation through continuity in cultural beliefs and attitudes was not supported in its original simple form: reality was very much more complicated. We would not wish to exaggerate the degree of health deprivation which we found, for there is no doubt that in this social group and this geographical area the advances made in child health during the fifty or so years covered by the lifetimes of the three generations have been outstanding. Nevertheless there must still be some cause for concern about the children of the present generation, and we hope that our detailed data may not only help to explain why health deprivation still occurs, but also help to suggest ways in which improvements can be made.

References
[1] Department of Health and Social Security (1980), *Inequalities in Health,* Report of a Working Party of the Chief Scientist Organisation, London: HMSO.

[2] Butler, N. R. and Alberman E. D. (eds.) (1969), *Perinatal Problems: the Second Report of the 1958 British Perinatal Mortality Survey*, Edinburgh: E. and S. Livingstone.
Brotherston, Sir J. (1976), 'Inequality: is it inevitable?' (The Galton Lecture) in Carter, C. O. and Peel, J. (eds.), *Equalities and Inequalities in Health*, London: Academic Press.
Blaxter, M. (1981), *The Health of the Children*, London: Heinemann Educational Books.

[3] Davie, R., Butler, N. and Goldstein H. (1972), *From Birth to Seven: the Second Report of the National Child Development Study (1958 Cohort)*, London: Longman.
Wedge, P. and Prosser, H. (1973), *Born to Fail?*, London: Arrow Books and the National Children's Bureau.
Court Report (1976), *Fit for the Future*, Report of the Committee on Child Health Services, Cmnd. 6684, London: HMSO.

[4] Davie *et al.* (1972), op. cit.

[5] Lewis, O. (1968), *La Vida*, London: Panther Books.

[6] Weeks, H. A., Davis, M. and Freeman, H. (1958), 'Apathy of families toward medical care: an exploratory study' in Jaco, E. G. (ed.) *Patients, Physicians and Illness*, Glencoe: Free Press.
Suchman, E. A. (1964), 'Socio-medical variations among ethnic groups', *Amer. J. Soc.*, **70**, 319.
Rainwater, L. (1968), 'The lower class: health, illness and medical institutions' in Deutscher, I. and Thompson, E. J. (eds.), *Among the People: Encounters with the Poor*, New York: Basic Books.
Kosa, J., Antonovsky, A. and Zola, I. K. (eds.) (1969), *Poverty and Health: a Sociological Analysis*, Cambridge, Mass.: Havard University Press.
Tongue W. L. (1975), 'Families without hope: a controlled study of 33

problem families', *Brit. J. Psychiat.*, Pubn. no. 11, London: Headley Bros.

[7] Rosengren, W. R. (1964), 'Social class and becoming ill' in Shostak, A. and Gomberg, W. (eds.), *Blue Collar World*, Englewood Cliffs, N.J.: Prentice-Hall.
Rosenblatt, D. and Suchman, E. A. (1964), 'Blue-collar attitudes and orientation toward health and illness' in Shostak, A. and Gomberg, W. (eds.), *Blue Collar World*, Englewood Cliffs, N.J.: Prentice-Hall.
Suchman, E. A. (1965), 'Social factors in medical deprivation', *Amer. J. Pub. Health*, **55**, 1725.
Osofsky, H. J. (1968), 'The walls are within: an exploration of barriers between middle-class physicians and poor patients' in Deutscher, I. and Thompson, E. J. (eds.), *Among the People: Encounters with the Poor*, New York: Basic Books.

[8] Rosenstock, I. M. (1969), 'Prevention of illness and maintenance of health' in Kosa, J., Antonovsky, A. and Zola, I. K. (eds.), *Poverty and Health: a Sociological Analysis*, Cambridge, Mass.: Harvard University Press.

[9] Leacock, E. G. (1971), *The Culture of Poverty: a Critique*. New York: Simon and Schuster.
Greenlick, M. R., Freeborn, D. K., Colombo, J. J., Prossin, J. A. and Saward, E. W. (1972), 'Comparing the use of medical care services by a medically indigent and a general membership population in a comprehensive prepaid group practice program', *Medical Care*, **10**, 187.
Valentine, C. A. (1968), *Culture and Poverty: Critique and Counter-Proposals*, Chicago: University of Chicago Press.

[10] Coburn, D. and Pope, C. R. (1974), 'Socioeconomic status and preventive health behaviour', *J. Health and Soc. Behav.*, **15**, 67.
Andersen, R., Kravits, J. and Anderson, O. W. (eds.) (1975), *Equity in Health Services: Empirical Analyses in Social Policy*, Cambridge, Mass.: Balinger.
Dutton, D. (1978), 'Explaining the low use of health services by the poor: costs, attitudes or delivery systems?', *Amer. Soc. Rev.*, **43**, 348.
Wan, T. H. and Gray, L. C. (1978), 'Differential access to preventive services for young children in low-income urban areas', *J. Health and Soc. Behav.*, **19**, 312.
Rundall, T. G. and Wheeler, J. R. C. (1979), 'The effect of income on the use of preventive care: an evaluation of alternative explanations', *J. Health and Soc. Behav.*, **20**, 397.

[11] Morris, N., Hatch, M. H. and Chapman, S. S. (1966), 'Deterrents to well-child supervision', *Amer. J. Pub. Health*, **56**, 1232.
Strauss, A. L. (1969), 'Medical organisation, medical care and lower income groups', *Soc. Sci. Med.*, **3**, 143.
McKinlay, J. B. (1972), 'Some approaches and problems in the study of the use of services', *J. Health and Soc. Behav.*, **13**, 115.
Antonovsky, A. (1972), 'A model to explain visits to the doctor', *J. Health and Soc. Behav.*, **13**, 446.

[12] McKinlay, J. B. and McKinlay, S. M. (1972), 'Some social characteristics of lower working class utilisers and under-utilisers of maternity care services', *J. Health and Soc. Behav.*, **13**, 369.
Davie *et al.* (1972), op. cit.

[13] Davie *et al.* (1972), op. cit.

[14] Court Report (1976), op. cit.

[15] Fabrega, H. (1977), 'The scope of ethnomedical science', *Culture, Medicine and Psychiatry*, **1**, 201.

[16] Litman, T. J. (1971), 'Health care and the family: a three-generational analysis', *Medical Care*, **9**, 67.

[17] Pratt, L. (1973), 'Child-rearing methods and children's health behaviour', *J. Health and Soc. Behav.*, **14**, 61.

[18] Sweetser, D. A. (1964), 'Mother–daughter ties between generations in industrial societies', *Process*, **3**, 332.
Litman, T. J. (1974), 'The family as a basic unit in health and medical care: a socio-behavioural overview', *Soc. Sci. and Med.*, **8**, 495.

[19] Mechanic, D. (1964), 'The influence of mothers on their children's health attitudes and behaviour', *Paediatrics*, **33**, 444.

[20] Litman, T. J. (1971), op. cit.

2   Method of the Study

The sample chosen for the examination of these issues consisted of 58 three-generation families. It was obviously not possible to consider both attitudes and behaviour in an intensive way in a large and random sample of families representing all the variables that might be relevant: social class and education, economic status and environment, geographical region and subculture, age and degree of close association between the generations. Therefore, the strategy was adopted of studying the 'most likely' case, choosing families who probably belonged to a close subculture and where it was known that continued contact between mother and married daughter was common.

The families all lived in one Scottish City, and had broadly the same structure of health services available to them. They were, by definition, neither geographically nor socially mobile. The older women, the *grandmother* generation, had borne their children in this city, and had at that time been in social classes IV or V, semi- or unskilled manual occupations. They still lived in the City. Their daughters, the *mother* generation, had also borne a child or children in the City, still lived there, and had been in the same social classes at the time of the last child's birth. It was amongst these families, if anywhere, that the 'transmission' of attitudes might be found. It was also among these families that one might expect to find some evidence of poorer health among children.

A note on the selection of the sample is included at Appendix A, and the social circumstances of the families are described in chapter 3. Some of them were indeed socially disturbed or in poor economic circumstances. It must be made clear, however, that they are certainly not defined *a priori* as a 'deprived' group. Though almost all of the young families remained in the same social classes, many were socially stable and economically secure. Comparisons will be made within the group between the more, and the less, disadvantaged families. The group as a whole is defined simply as a working-class group, located within a particular subculture and environment, in a range of socioeconomic circumstances.

Data Collection

The phenomena being examined are of several different sorts. We wished to study, and if possible to make connections between, the health histories and social histories of the families, the attitudes and beliefs of each generation, the health-related behaviour and health-service use of the young mothers, and the actual health experience of the children. The topics thought to be relevant, besides general concepts of health and orientations towards medicine, included family-building behaviour, antenatal care, preventive behaviour, accidents, nutrition, the use of lay remedies and lay advice, and many others. Several different methods of data collection, used in combination, therefore seemed most fruitful.

(1) Firstly, the co-operation of the young mothers was sought for a longitudinal study of the health and health-service use of the children over six months in each family. At monthly visits, the women were asked to report any symptoms which their children had experienced during the past four weeks, and to talk about the actions taken, the advice sought, and the services used. From these accounts we attempted to establish at what level of symptomology the mother perceived that ill health existed, and at what level of ill health she took action of what sort. Thus, a picture of the children's health over six months can be presented, though the focus is not so much upon actual morbidity as upon response to illness and utilisation of services. Interaction with other services besides general practitioners—dentists, health visitors, social workers, child health clinics, specialist clinics, children's hospital, school health services—was also recorded.

The reliability of these data will be discussed in the relevant sections, but in general we believe them to be reasonably complete and accurate. The use of the technique of health diaries had been considered, but we believe it would have been successful in only a proportion of the families.

(2) On an initial visit to each young mother, information was obtained about her own health and her husband's, her education, working and married life, and her perception of her children's general health and health history. During the six-months' survey period this information was supplemented by wide-ranging discussions of different aspects of health-related behaviour, emotional, financial and housing problems, relationships with grandparents, friends and neighbours, and many other topics relevant to the upbringing of the children. Our own observation during the regular and often lengthy visits, though necessarily limited, was also sometimes useful.

(3) Obviously, we can be less sure of the accuracy of the data on the children's health history than on the events at the present time, since the accounts may cover many years and are likely to have been rewritten, at least to some extent, in the respondent's memory. We were, however, able to examine various records concerning the children (maternity, child health clinic, pre-school assessment, health visiting) in order to compare them with the mother's accounts. From these records information could be extracted on each child's birth condition, 'At Risk' status, accounts of illness, injury and development problems during each year of the child's life, assessments of home conditions, immunisation records and the results of routine screening. Also, after the six-months' survey was completed, the health visitor who was in contact with each family was interviewed. We discussed with them the general health of the children and the health care provided by the mother, and explored their view of their role in helping these young families. For events occurring during the survey period, we were also able to compare the perceptions of the mother and the health visitor about what had happened.

(4) Data of a different sort, concerned with the attitudes of the women of each generation, their norms, values, beliefs and perceptions of past and present structures of health services, were obtained by interviews which were usually tape-recorded and lasted from one to three hours. The interview with the mother, at the conclusion of the six months, included a discussion of the events that had been reported, and a more general review of ideas about health. The interview with the grandmother focused upon her health and health history, her own childbearing and child-rearing practices, and her attitudes to illness, doctors, and health services. Since not all grandmothers agreed to be interviewed, there are 47 of these interviews.

(5) We have, of course, no independent data on the health behaviour or health-service use of the older generation at the present time. Advantage was taken, however, of the existence of extensive information from a study of women of this generation at the time of their first delivery in 1950–53, followed up five and ten years later.[1] At that time 455 women (of all social classes) had been studied, though only a small number could be traced who now filled the requirements for the present sample. Thirty of our 47 grandmothers are in fact from the original study. For these women, their current presentation can be compared with the information which was recorded in the 1950–53 study, on such topics as family planning, antenatal care, living conditions, marital relationships, and the health of their children during the early years. It may perhaps be of

interest to note that though there were a few topics on which the women's memory was faulty, or they preferred to be vague (e.g. attendance at antenatal or child health clinics), the accuracy of the information on most subjects, after twenty-five to thirty years, was surprising.

The Nature of the Data

It will be obvious that two very different types of data are being used in this study: on the one hand, 'factual' information about the health of the children and about health-related behaviour in the young families, and on the other, data of a different sort, concerned with attitudes and perceptions. It is suggested that both types are useful, and that a combination of them is essential if explanations are to be sought. We wished to ascertain facts as reliably as possible, and at the same time to explore the meaning of these facts to the individuals concerned, attempting to offer explanations for their behaviour in terms of their perception of events. Since different methods of analysis are appropriate for different sorts of data, the variety of methods used in succeeding chapters is a deliberate attempt to apply several different techniques to particular aspects of the same subject.

These methods do not include the categorisation of health or the measurement of attitudes by means of structured questionnaire. There is a research tradition of measuring concepts such as 'medical fatalism' or 'medical orientation' by the scored agreement or dis-agreement with abstract or hypothetical statements such as 'People have no control over whether they become sick or not'[2] or 'I have my doubts about some things doctors say they can do for you',[3] and to describe self-perceived health by the answers to checklists of symptoms. With large studies, such methods may be necessary. It has, however, frequently been shown that the recognition of one's own ill health in a structured list may be problematic: 'People fail to recognise their rheumatism in a question about swollen and painful joints'[4] and that

> For many people there seems to be a frame of reference . . . that may only be discovered either by giving them carte blanche to talk about their health or by using exactly their own terminology.[5]

The intention in this study was therefore not to impose a frame of reference upon the respondents, nor to apply preconceived categories or concepts of 'health' or 'disease'. Rather, the women's words were examined to discover their own terminologies, and their models of sickness, ideas about disease, and views of health services were derived from the transcripts of their conversations.

All interviews were semi-structured, i.e. based on a list of topics to be covered or items of information to be obtained, but adapted in each case to the individual history and situation. For instance, generalised questions such as 'What do you think about medical science?' were as far as possible avoided; instead, the question to the older women might be, 'You say you have this arthritis, do you think they'll ever find a cure for it? Is this true of most things?' In a similar way, the mothers were encouraged to talk about the reported incidents concerning the child's health.

The attitudes displayed may well be multi-dimensional and not necessarily consistent, of course; people may hold incompatible beliefs concurrently, or express different attitudes in different contexts. We hope that the analysis allows for this. Nor are the histories given, the accounts of illnesses in the past, or the reports of what happened during interactions with doctors, necessarily factually correct. It is the woman's story, true or false, which represents her perception of the social fact of sickness, and it is on this that attitudes are based.

We were fully aware that the survey situation itself might affect the nature of the accounts which were given, and might even affect the behaviour of the young mothers. Despite attempts to guard against this by taking a completely neutral stand on all the topics which were discussed, it is probable that some contamination did occur. For example, after comparing the behaviour during the survey with the previous behaviour noted on health-visitor or clinic cards, it appears likely that a few women were prompted to take their children for immunisation or assessment, to specialist clinics and to general practitioners, when they might otherwise not have done so. This perceived influence is noted in the relevant sections.

Presentation
After a description of the families, and a general discussion of concepts of health and illness, each aspect of the children's health and the mothers' health-care behaviour is dealt with first in a quantified and factual way, and then by a more descriptive or ethnographic treatment of the mothers' perception of these events.

Throughout, there are many direct quotations from the respondents, who can often speak most eloquently for themselves. All material which is in quotation marks, or set off from the rest of the text, is directly quoted from transcripts or verbatim notes. To identify the families and individuals, the grandmother in each family is referred to as G1, G2, G3, etc. and the mother as M1, M2, M3, etc. The reader is thus able, if he wishes, to identify the material which refers to the same family in different sections, to relate mothers to grandmothers, and to compare different quotations from the same individual. Exceptions are made only in a few cases where it seemed better, in the interests of confidentiality, to avoid this linking. Of course, every care has been taken to avoid the possibility that any family or individual could be recognised.

References

[1] Thompson, B. and Illsley, R. (1969), 'Family growth in Aberdeen', *J. Biosocial Sci.*, **1**, 23.

[2] Mechanic, D. (1964), 'The influence of mothers on their children's health attitudes and behaviour', *Paediatrics*, **33**, 444.

[3] Suchman, E. A. (1965), 'Social factors in medical deprivation', *Amer. J. Public Health*, **55**, 1725.

[4] Cartwright, A. (1959), 'Some problems in the collection and analysis of morbidity data obtained from sample surveys', *Milbank Mem. Fund. Quart.*, **41**, 1.

[5] Wadsworth, M. E. J., Butterfield, W. J. H. and Blaney, R. (1971), *Health and Sickness: the Choice of Treatment*, London: Tavistock.

3 The Sample Families

In this chapter a brief description is given of the social history and present circumstances of the sample families, in order to provide a background to the succeeding chapters.

The Grandmothers

The average age of the 47 grandmothers interviewed was 51 years. Most of them had thus been born about 1930, and begun their families in the early 1950s. Their husbands had at that time all been in semi-skilled or unskilled jobs, and many were described as having been in poorly paid or insecure work, or had frequent periods of unemployment. Roughly a fifth of the husbands had been trawlermen or merchant seamen. Most of the women had been themselves brought up in this City, in which they had lived all their life; about a quarter of them, however, described rural childhoods, often in farm-labouring families, and a later migration to the City.

For many, their own childhoods in pre-war days had been very hard. Almost all had left school at 14 and gone out to work. The description of one was:

> My mother had ten altogether, six of us survived. I was brought up wi' my grandparents. My grandmother died when I was eight. I went to stay with my mother from then until I was almost thirteen when she died. That's when we lost her. I kept the family together for six months, on my own, at that age—goin' to school as well—until we got someone to take us all. And then I left school at 14 and went out to work on the farms.(G30)

Table 3.1 *Number of children born to grandmothers (completed families) and mothers (up to the present time)*

	Number of children										
	1	*2*	*3*	*4*	*5*	*6*	*7*	*8*	*9*	*12*	*Total*
Number of grandmothers	2	12	9	8	8	3	2	—	2	1	47
Number of mothers	4	29	20	5	—	—	—	—	—	—	58

Note: In the case of the younger generation, the total number of children is 142 rather than the 139 children who are in this survey. The three additional children are illegitimate children not living with the present families.

The women married at an average age of 21, and bore their first child at an average age of 22. Their mean family size was four children, and their family sizes are set beside those of their daughters, the mother generation, in Table 3.1. Of the 30 women on whom 1950–53 data are available, over half had conceived their first child prenuptially.[1]

The early childbearing years of these women were described as little more prosperous than their own childhoods. Subletting of one crowded room from their parents or other relatives was common when they were first married. A proportion had occupied local authority property, but it had usually been poor pre-war tenements in notoriously 'bad' areas. The remainder had rented rooms, often overcrowded or damp, with no bathroom, frequently no running water, and commonly an outside toilet. One woman described it thus:

> We were three years married, we were living with my husband's mother. There were no houses at that time, you were lucky if you got a room. Working-class folks buying houses at that time, well that was just unheard of. Five pounds was the average wage, you see, for someone labouring an' that. There just wasn't work at the time—and in the wintertime, 'I think I'll have my books tomorrow', or 'bound to get them next week'—we were born too early! See what they get now! (G37)

Only a handful of the women presented themselves as being free from money problems. At least a third described severe financial difficulties in their early married years, and the rest had to manage their incomes carefully. They saw this, and the better housing, as the main difference between their daughters' lives and their own.

> We didn't have the money in those days, did we—they can do a lot more for children now than what we could ever do. We had to go to jumble sales for clothes, but they can *buy* them and that sort of thing now. (G32)

There were few complaints about early poverty, though. Indeed, many women struggled to reconcile their feeling—common in an older generation looking back, of course—that family life was better in the past, with their knowledge that their daughters were very much less disadvantaged:

> Let's face it, life's a lot easier than it ever wis—the good old days wis harder days for us. But you wis happier—nowadays you're gettin' mair money but you canna dee the same wi' it ... That's the livin' gone oot o' life, isn't it? I've had a lot mair than they'll ever get—and I niver got nuthin'! Little things that counted in our time. It's the big things that disnae count in this time. (G19)

Nor did those women, now, dwell on their disturbed social history, though they did not conceal it either. From their matter-of-fact stories, and from the records available from the earlier period, it was clear that the earlier years of childbearing in the 1950s had been, for many, a troubled period. There was a proportion of husbands who had been drinkers and violent towards their families, and in at least seven of the 30 families on whom there were data from 1950-53, there were records of serious assaults, the desertion of the family by husband or wife, or children placed in care.

These dramatic troubles must not be exaggerated, however, since the majority of families struggled on quietly and contentedly. The past was often rosily remembered as a time of great contentment:

This going awa' oot—onything's an excuse for a night oot—when we wis young we didnae hae that kinda money, so we sorta contented oorsels, ken? I used to say to mysel' when the dark nights come in, 'Oh, that's fine, that, I like the dark nights', 'cos the kids were all in the hoose an' it wis fine.(G31)

Despite their financial hardships, work outside the home had not been universal for the women in the 1950s, and had not been considered desirable. The work available to most of these women had generally been unskilled, part-time, poorly paid and frequently unpleasant, for few had educational attainment or skills to offer. Fish processing, cleaning, part-time factory and shop work were common. The widowed, separated and divorced and the wives of the unemployed were, of course, often forced to take full-time employment, despite the problems of child care which were presented.

Since these early days of marriage the situation of the 'grand-mother' generation had changed considerably, however. Of the 47 interviewed, 11 were now widowed, three had been widowed and remarried, and four were divorced or separated, one for the second time.

The majority now appeared to be financially secure. Although many of their husbands, if still alive, were still in semi-skilled or unskilled occupations, their jobs were now secure and settled. With most of their children now independent, not only did the families have fewer financial commitments, but the women were also more free to work. There were also more, and more pleasant, jobs available. Approximately a quarter of the women now worked full-time, typically in shops, offices, or as auxiliary nurses. Most of the rest had some part-time work, of a more satisfying nature (for instance, hospital domestic work) than in the past.

Their environment had also improved dramatically. Few remained in the worst local authority flats, and most were now in modern blocks or in semi-detached or terraced council houses, in pleasant areas. Two owned their own homes.

Health history

The 47 women who were interviewed were encouraged to talk about health and illness in the days of their own childhood, and were asked if they remembered the advent of the National Health Service (NHS). The memories that many had of the years before the war—with tuberculosis rife, and diphtheria or scarlet fever sweeping through whole families—illustrated vividly the very real advances of the last thirty or forty years. The early death of parents had been a commonplace, and the women made a clear connection between the environment of their childhood and the likelihood of disease. On the other hand, this involved some conflict with their wish to present the days of their youth as 'healthier', with simpler 'good food', fresh air, and sensible living: it was sometimes preferable, therefore, to attribute the disappearance of the diseases responsible for early deaths in the past to the advance of medical science, rather than to improvements in living conditions:

> I always had sore throats, septic throats and that. Before I had diphtheria we stayed in an old house . . . my mother blamed that. We'd only one room and there was six o' us in one room, two beds in one room at that time. An' your sink was just in the stair an' outside wis your toilet. But they've cured this diphtheria now, you dinna hardly hear aboot it.(G3)

This recollection of pre-NHS days varied. About a third could not remember their parents paying for treatment or using the 'parish' doctor for the poor, or did not discuss the subject at all. Over half did remember their parents paying or being 'on the parish', though they did not associate the memories with any severe deprivation of health care. Some of those who themselves had young children in pre-NHS days talked of the period in a matter-of-fact fashion: yes, they had to pay, it was extremely difficult, but they had found the money somehow. The advent of the NHS was nevertheless memorable:

> You knew a difference efter that. I mean to say, we called up wur ain doctor then, and didnae hae the worry of paying bills. I mind once I had a thirteen shillin' bill to pay. At that time thirteen shillin's was a fortune. I'd got it paid some way or other. It must have been some o' the bairns nae weel—at night, when you'd to call a private doctor.(G15)

A small number of the women did, however, remember severe hardship in the days before the NHS:

> My mother—she wis bothered wi' kidney trouble, forty years ago—an' payin' for the doctor, an' she had the three of us—she jist couldnae afford the doctor an' just sorta put up wi' it. She put off goin' to the doctor until she's now in a wheelchair. If it had been now, she wouldn't hae been in the state she's in now.(G25)

In some cases, they attributed their own chronic conditions similarly to lack of medical care:

> When you had to pay for a doctor? Well—to this day my mother still says that was the reason that I took rheumatic fever. 'Cos I took scarlet fever—and I was ill for a few days, and my mother took me to the dispensary... Now, I had to walk there, 'cos my mother didn't have the tram-car fare. With the result—I got my chill—we had to walk to the dispensary because it was free there, we couldn't afford to pull in a doctor. 'Cos my mother would have had the doctor in her house—well, at least twice a week because she had eight of us.(G1)

We have, of course, no independent data on the health of this generation at the present time. From their accounts, however—and these are by definition survivors—this early history and in some cases neglect had resulted in a high prevalence of chronic conditions. Table 3.2 presents a list of all the more serious or chronic diseases which the 47 women mentioned, necessarily relying upon their own

Table 3.2 Chronic conditions reported by 47 women of the 'grandmother' generation (with number of women, if more than one)

Bronchitis (13)	Gynaecological problems (10)
Rheumatism (3)	Menopausal syndrome (4)
Arthritis (5)	Tuberculosis (skin, not active)
Sciatica (2)	Breast cancer (not active)
Stroke (2)	Congenital syphilis
Asthma (5)	Stomach trouble, ulcers (3)
Anaemia	Overweight (treated) (5)
Deafness (3)	Gallbladder trouble (3)
'Brittle bones'	High blood pressure (2)
Pancreatitis	Heart disease (3)
Swollen ankles, bad circulation (3)	Varicose veins (2)
Kidney disease, 'bladder trouble',	Thyroid trouble
chronic cystitis (4)	Partial sight (2)
Tuberculosis (pulmonary, not active) (5)	Dermatitis (for 34 years)
Back trouble, spine trouble, slipped disc (8)	'Anxiety neurosis' (psychiatrically
'Nerves', depression (psychiatrically treated) (4)	treated)
Migraine, chronic headache (6)	

reported diagnoses. Some of these, of course, may be mistaken, and there were also vague, undiagnosed complaints. The list is certainly incomplete. It can be noted that these women had, at the time of interview, an average of more than two of these conditions each. The social and medical history which has been briefly described is obviously very relevant to the discussion of attitudes to health which follows in subsequent chapters.

The Mothers

The childhood years of the next generation, the daughters of these women, had typically been spent in the poor housing of their mothers' younger days, and some had been brought up in disturbed and broken families. Of the 30 families for which 1950–53 data could be consulted, all but four were subletting rooms from parents or other relatives at the time when these women were born. Only one girl attended a selective (grammar) school (this was for a brief period only), and all but a few left school at the minimum age. Their average age at marriage was 19, and the average age at first delivery just over 19. (Table 3.3 shows the mothers' age at first delivery.) Nineteen of the children within the present survey families were illegitimate; 15 were born before marriage, and four were not the present husband's child. Five women had pregnancies terminated before marriage and one miscarried. Thirty-four of the live births within marriage were prenuptial conceptions; 11 of the women with no prenuptially conceived live children already had an illegitimate child or termination before marriage. Four women had terminations, and 13 had miscarriages, after marriage. Seven women had an illegitimate child and then conceived prenuptially, two had an illegitimate child *and* a termination before marriage, and there was a variety of other patterns.

The average family size of the sample is 2.4 and the women on average had a space of 2.6 years between their first and second child but Table 3.4 shows that only one or two years was most common. There was an average of 2.5 years between the second and third child, and in the four families with four children 1.5 years between third and fourth.

The social circumstances of the young women had sometimes been very difficult in the earliest childbearing years, especially for those with youthful pregnancies and illegitimate children. There were those who at that time had been disowned by their parents, or on the other hand had experienced deep conflict with a mother who wanted to bring up an illegitimate grandchild herself. One woman described her days as a young single-handed parent as 'up at 6, baby to nursery

Table 3.3 Mothers' age at first delivery

	Age of mother										
	16	17	18	19	20	21	22	23	24	25	Total
Number of mothers	4	7	16	14	6	2	3	3	2	1	58

Table 3.4 Years between first and second child

	Years								Total
	1	2	3	4	5	6	7	8	
Number of mothers	15	15	11	4	6	—	1	1	53

Note: The three children not living within the present families are excluded.

at 7, work at 8, my sister babysitting so I could do overtime, weekends to do housework'.

Nor had the marriages of many been without difficulties. Four women were divorced or legally separated, and living as 'single parents' during the six months; two of them reported that they had been assaulted by their ex-husbands. Four women were divorced and since remarried; two were known to have been abused by their first husbands, and one regularly beaten by her second. Health visitors suggested that three other women had been assaulted by their husbands, but these mothers did not reveal this during our interviews. The records of two of the women showed that they had previously attempted to stab their partner; these couples were still together, albeit in a stormy or violent relationship.

One husband and one wife left home during the research period. A further ten women openly admitted that their marriages were or had been unhappy, with periods of separation and severe conflict. In sum, 23 of the mothers were believed to have experienced a troubled married life. At least five of the fathers had prison records, in some cases for crimes of violence.

This disturbed picture must not, of course, be extended to the whole sample. The majority of marriages—about two-thirds of the current marriages—were at least without obvious conflict, and many of these appeared to be loving and stable relationships.

The housing and other circumstances of the young families at the time of the survey were much more diverse and difficult to typify than their mothers' had been. They had occupied their present home for an average of four years; some had lived there as long as nine years, while others had recently moved. Very few women went straight into their present home on marriage. Half of the sample previously sublet a room from a mother or mother-in-law; most were overcrowded since they generally had a baby soon afterwards. Seven families had one spell in private rented accommodation, often cramped, damp and lacking basic amenities. Twelve families had two homes before moving into their present one—usually a variety of sublets, privately rented rooms, council flats and caravans. Six women had three or more varied moves, with one woman claiming to have made as many as 14.

The great majority now lived in council flats of various types and ages, whilst the remaining few occupied local authority terraced or semi-detached housing. Only one family was buying their own home. About a third lived in the worst areas, where the surroundings are bleak, 'gardens' are communal expanses of mud, and vandalism is rife; about a quarter lived in intermediate areas and the remainder in quite pleasant surroundings. However, housing area does not necessarily correlate with housing standard, since good houses were found in the poorest areas and vice versa. Thirteen families inhabited housing which we judged to be of a poor standard (e.g. damp, in a bad state of repair), and a further 19 occupied homes which were structurally mediocre; the rest of the housing was of an acceptable standard.

Ten of the families were judged to be 'overcrowded', defined as more than two persons per bedroom. In five of the homes the furnishings and equipment seemed inadequate, and in a further 16, adequate but very basic. Seven homes were regularly very untidy and dirty; the housekeeping standards of a further eight families were judged to be 'indifferent', but we must acknowledge the difficult task of mothers with many small children running and crawling around. All these housing factors were taken into account in the index of 'disadvantage' described in Appendix B.

About a fifth of the families appeared to be experiencing considerable financial difficulties, living at the level of Family Income Supplement or Supplementary Benefit. A similar number were just managing to cope, often with assistance from relatives, while the remainder seemed to be fairly comfortable. However, among many of the families financial circumstances fluctuated dramatically with occupational changes.

The sample was chosen on the basis that the husband was noted in maternity records as having a semi-skilled or unskilled manual occupation at the time of the most recent child's birth (not including children born during the study). Since that time, however, there had been a certain amount of occupational change. Considering occupation when in work, and the ex-husband's occupation of the divorced, 33 men were unskilled manual workers in the building trade, fish processing, oil rigs and so on; 12 men were semi-skilled, for example factory workers, drivers in warehouses, etc.; a further 12 were skilled manual workers such as panel beaters, bricklayers, painters, etc., and one father had been promoted to a non-manual post in a firm for which he had worked for many years. Unlike the men of the previous generation, none of the husbands were trawler-men though one father left the sea, before the study began, because of ill health. These families demonstrated clearly that conventional classifications of social class may be problematic in this particular age and social group, and in this area. The arbitrary nature of occupational categories is shown by the fact that one husband was a painter, labourer, bus driver, oil-rig worker and 'personnel manager' all within a fairly short time, and others had similar if not quite such dramatic changes. Some men habitually did different types of work in winter and summer, or moved to any type of work that would command a better wage.

Two of the husbands were Registered Disabled and this severely limited the employment opportunities of one of them. A further ten men had medical conditions, such as stomach ulcers or back trouble, which necessitated prolonged sickness absence during the six months; three were in fact off work for most of the time. Due to the nature of their work several men sustained industrial injuries, and there was evidence that several fathers drank rather heavily. Nine men had a period of unemployment during the six months, or drifted in and out of work; two were unemployed for the whole period. Ten husbands had spells working away from home, primarily in connection with the oil industry.

Before marriage, approximately one quarter of the women worked in an office. Ten girls worked in factories, primarily paper mills, ten worked in shops, eight in textile mills and six in fish processing. The less common pre-marital occupations included hairdressing and cleaning. Now, like their mothers before them, they found it difficult or undesirable to be employed outside the home. Twenty-three women did not work at all. Nine worked full-time at some time during the six months in the sorts of jobs outlined above; in these cases the children were school or nursery age and/or cared for by a grandmother or unemployed husband. The majority of the other mothers cleaned, worked in fish processing, bars or restaurants in the evenings, or during the day if they could arrange for the super-vision of the children for a few hours.

Twenty-four of the women lived a short walking distance from their mother's (or mother-in-law's) home, sometimes in the same block of flats or street. Sixteen needed a short bus trip or a long walk in order to visit granny; a further 18 families were separated by greater distance, e.g. a longer bus trip or two separate journeys. However, geographical problems did not deter most of the women, who would struggle on to buses with several small children in order to visit 'mum'. In other cases granny would attempt the journey, or they would meet at some convenient mid-way point such as a relative's house or a shopping area. As a result 28 women saw their mother every day or almost every day, and all but a few of the others met on average once or twice a week.

Health history

There are documented data on their early health history, from the 1950–53 study, for only half the mothers. The health records and assessments which were carried out at five years of age often note a clear connection between infant ill health and the economically deprived, and often disturbed, early married days which were typical of the grandmother generation. Not all the mother generation were adversely affected, of course: for perhaps a third, the earlier records note that, as children, they were 'surprisingly healthy given the appalling lack of facilities', 'a revelation' considering 'the conditions in this typical slum family', or 'a credit to a conscientious mother'. The majority of this group of the mother generation, however, had suffered before they were five from conditions such as bronchitis, pneumonia, jaundice, dysentery, and gastroenteritis. Measles, mumps and whooping cough had been very common. There were many records of accidents, and enuresis was very frequently mentioned. The examining doctors of the five-year olds had also been particularly concerned about lack of dental care, describing the majority of the children as having 'neglected and carious' teeth, and some as exhibiting 'only blackened stumps'.

To this record must be added many serious illnesses in their childhood described by the grandmother generation. This cannot, however, be regarded as a complete or reliable account, since (as described in chapter 4) the grandmothers were very apt to describe the children as 'healthy', and to mention much of the ill health of the past only incidentally.

The health of the mother generation now, as young women in their 20s, varied: some presented themselves as experiencing very little ill health, but in general there was a high prevalence of certain chronic conditions. They cannot be directly compared with their mothers, of course, for the middle-aged group might be expected to report more chronic diseases. Their daughters did not have so long a history to talk about, nor was the subject of health such an interesting one for

Table 3.5   Chronic conditions reported by 58 women of the 'mother' generation (with number of women, if more than one)

Bronchitis, 'bad chest', 'lung infections' (7)	Asthma (3)
Tuberculosis (not active) (2)	Chronic cough (2)
Kidney disease, chronic cystitis (10)	Stomach trouble (2)
Gallbladder trouble (5)	Chronic constipation (2)
Gynaecological problems (9)	Anaemia (8)
Diabetes (3)	'Back trouble' (2)
Sinus trouble (2)	Migraine, chronic headache (3)
'Trouble with legs', varicose veins (3)	Hare lip (repaired)
Overweight (treated) (6)	Partial deafness
Skin disease, eczema (2)	Partial sight (2)
Depression, 'nerves' (psychiatrically treated) (2)	

them. Nevertheless, as Table 3.5 shows, a large number of chronic diseases were reported at some time during the six-months' contact with the young families.

As with the older generation, chest diseases, overweight, and gynaecological problems were particularly common. Gynaecological trouble and bladder problems were very often held to be the result of childbearing. Although the number of conditions reported by the young women is—as might be expected—less than that reported by their mothers, nevertheless the record seemed poor for a group still in their 20s. One of the young women expressed her feelings about her own health status very clearly:

> Like, other folk, you say to yourself 'There's never anything the matter with them.' But when you get older, like my mother's age, I think they start getting things like—like gallbladder or something like that—you sort of expect things when you get older. I feel like, I'm only 26 and I say to myself 'Oh, I'm only young', you know. And sometimes I feel like I'm maybe 56 . . . you've got three young kids and you say to yourself 'It's nae real, this.' It makes you depressed.(M1)

The Children
Table 3.6 shows that all but two of the 139 children of the families were nine years old and younger at the time of the survey. Two of the children shown as less than one year were in fact babies born during the survey.

Sixty-two of the children were attending school at the commencement of the survey period; several others, of course, joined them during the six months. Table 3.7 shows the numbers of pre-school and school children in the sample.

Table 3.6   Distribution of ages of children in the sample

					Age, years							
	⟨1	1	2	3	4	5	6	7	8	9	10	11	Total
Number of children													
Male	9	3	8	11	8	9	8	7	3	2	—	1	69
Female	3	6	13	8	8	5	6	5	9	6	1	—	70
													139

Table 3.7   Numbers of pre-school and school children in the sample

	Pre-school, not at nursery	Part-time or full-time nursery school	Primary school	Special school
Numbers of children				
Male	23	16	28	2
Female	25	13	32	—

A considerable proportion of the pre-school children of three and four years old attended nursery school, the majority attending part-time the nursery section of the local primary school, though a few had secured private or full-time local authority provision. A policy of positive discrimination in certain areas of the City appeared to be in operation, although a few mothers in one pocket of housing did experience some difficulty. Several of the children had been given 'priority' places, because (for instance) of the mother's mental state, because the mother worked full-time while the father was unemployed, or because of persistent accidents or behaviour problems.

References
[1] Women with illegitimate children were excluded from the 1950–53 study, so that the proportion of the grandmother generation derived from that study are not entirely representative of all social class IV and V women bearing children at the time.

4 Concepts of Health, Illness and Disease

The social history and characteristics which have been described may obviously be expected to affect the concepts of health, illness and disease held by this group of women. It is necessary to distinguish the three concepts, and they will be dealt with in turn.

The distinction between 'illness' and 'disease' is one which is commonly made in medical sociology. Field,[1] for instance, points out that disease 'refers to a medical conception of pathological abnormality... indicated by a set of signs and symptoms', and illness 'refers primarily to a person's experience of ill health and is indicated by the person's feelings of pain, discomfort and the like'. He notes that it is possible to feel ill without having a disease, or to have a disease without feeling ill. Similarly, Fabrega[2] has discussed the fact that disease is independent of social behaviour, while illness is culturally-specific, dependent upon folk definitions of normality which may or may not have any relation to biomedical definitions, and has moral, psychological and social dimensions as well as physical. As Eisenberg[3] has summarised: 'Patients suffer illness: physicians diagnose and treat disease.'

The concept of health is more problematic. The oft-quoted World Health Organisation definition as 'a state of complete physical, mental and social well-being, not merely the absence of disease or infirmity' has been criticised as static and impossibly perfectionist,[4,5] and various definitions in terms of functional fitness have been suggested.[6,7]

The meaning of these concepts in various societies has been much studied by anthropologists, but how they are actually used by individuals in different social groups has not very often been investigated in developed societies. One notable exception is Herzlich's[8] study of the ideas of a group of Parisian women. The following discussion about the attitudes of this very different group in Scotland is derived, in part, from the responses of both older and younger generations to a set of rather general questions such as 'How has your health been over the years?' 'Do you feel that some people are naturally healthier than others?' or 'Would you say that your children are specially healthy or unhealthy?' In addition, all spontaneous mentions of health, illness or disease were extracted from the transcripts and interview notes for analysis, and each woman's set of expressed attitudes was examined for its form and logic.

Attitudes to Health

One important theme of the literature on the concept of 'health' is to point out that health may be understood in two ways: as a more or less static state of being, where to be healthy is to be in good structural and anatomical condition; or as a description of ongoing function, where to be healthy is to be able to carry out one's normal roles.[9] To be 'sick' or to feel 'ill' can be compatible with the first, but health in the second sense is the obverse of illness. Thus one may be 'unhealthy' in the first sense—crippled, diabetic, obese—and at the same time 'healthy' in the second—not ill, able to carry on living in a normal way. In both senses, of course, health is relative to personal or social norms. Health as a state of bodily functioning invokes higher expectations in the young than in the elderly, and people accommodate chronic conditions into their normal state.

The conventional greeting 'How are you?' calls forth a conventional reply in terms of the second definition of health: if they do not feel (abnormally) ill, people reply 'Very well', not 'As a matter of fact, I suffer from diabetes.' The extreme example of this is a paraplegic, replying to an interviewer in a study of disabled people 'Very well, thank-you—I've never been better.'[10]

Our questions to the respondents in this survey about their health may, to begin with, simply have tapped this same response. Despite the poor health records which have been described, by far the greater proportion of the older generation categorised their health and that of their families as 'good'. The younger generation were equally apt to reply 'good' or at least 'average'. As the interviews progressed, however, it became obvious that both generations tended to think of health *only* in the second sense of not ill, or able to carry on normally. This concept of health as a description of function was sustained with consistency throughout the interviews, and any questions which invited replies in terms of static state or condition were obviously found difficult to answer.

Indeed, the older generation, flying in the face of all the evidence (and they had talked about the ill health of the past in great detail), tended to resort to conventional presentations of a golden age of the past. Yes, there had of course been diseases rampant then which now had disappeared, and yes, illness had been caused by poverty and hardship, but—especially for those with rural backgrounds—nevertheless life had been in some sense healthier. Two examples are:

> My father didnae work frae during the first war—he was hurt in the war, so my mother had to bring up eight of us—it wis jist a case o' us getting—we got wur soup, we didnae get the best o' everything, we jist got the cheapest o' everything, but it wis a' *good*. I suppose that would give us a' the chance of better health.(G15)
> I think country people are far healthier than the townspeople are. We lived off the land, more or less . . . you're up early in the mornin', your work's not finished until maybe late at night, plenty o' fresh air . . . (G30)

Indeed, one of the grandmothers even managed to turn the prevalence of infectious disease into an advantage for health:

> O' course, measles affected your eyes. If the light got into your eyes you were blinded. But they thrive efter that. Efter they have the whooping cough an' measles an' that, then they thrive better.(G3)

The norms of what constituted good health, now, were conspicuously low. Good health was being able to work, being healthy enough 'for all practical purposes', not being admitted to hospital, having no 'big operations'. One woman, who had had tuberculosis and continued to suffer from bronchitis, still maintained that her health was reasonable because 'I'm a' right. I canna grumble—I've aye been able to go about an' that.' (G7)

Another, talking of her husband, said:

> He got part o' his lung taken oot. But he wis aye healthy enough. There wis niver nothin' the matter wi' him. (G31)

The younger generation were not quite so likely to describe themselves and their children as essentially healthy despite an eventful record of illness, but like their mothers they defined health in terms of not having illnesses, rather than in positive terms of fitness or unimpaired physique. One said of her husband:

> I suppose he would be really healthy because he's never been ill—cracked ribs, ulcer, things like that. But not a cold or 'flu.(M19)

and another of her daughter:

> She has trouble with her ears, but it's not actually her general health. It's extra to health.(M39)

The norms of the majority continued to be low. One, whose daughter had suffered recurrent ear infections, scarlet fever, and coughs said that she had 'never had a day's illness' and another, with one child who was crippled and others with chronic conditions, described them as 'very healthy children'. Healthy children were those who were never kept off school, or for brief periods only, or at least managed to be active: 'At least they can get out to play when ither eens can't.'(M30) It was inevitable that all children would be ill at some time: 'You can catch things even if you're healthy'(M41), but healthy children were less susceptible and caught fewer infectious diseases. M31, whose son suffered from convulsions, described him as 'definitely healthy' because 'he's not prone to take things'. Healthy children did not have 'right', 'real' or 'serious' illnesses, and in particular avoided chest complaints.

The ability to go to work had great symbolic importance: if one could work, or was not forced frequently to stay off work, then one must have good health. These low norms and tendency to define health only in functional terms can be illustrated by one longer example:

> After I was sterilised I had a lot of cystitis, and backache, because of the fibroids. Then when I had the hysterectomy I had bother wi' my waterworks because my bladder lived a life of its own and I had to have a repair . . . Healthwise I would say I'm OK. I did hurt my shoulder—I mean, this is nothing to do with health but I actually now have a disability, I get a gratuity payment every six months . . . I wear a collar and take Valium . . . then, just the headaches—but I'm not really off work a lot with it.(G29)

There was little evidence, in either generation, of health as a positive concept, a sense of well-being or physical fitness, and few took any steps to promote it. Indeed, there was a feeling that taking positive preventive or health-promoting action was 'cranky':

> You'll find a' this health-food fanatics an' keep-fit fanatics nae ony healthier than a person that just does their normal—their normal work, normal meals.(G40)
> I remember bein' in the Maternity an' watchin' them a' deein' exercises—and they says 'Come on now, Mrs B.' I says 'Away an' dinna annoy me, I niver did exercises in my life.'(G14)

Despite an extremely high rate of bronchial disease in the group, almost all the women smoked. Although one or two paid lip-service to health education slogans about cigarettes being detrimental to health, most of the women claimed they were entirely unconvinced by 'the statistics' or 'rumours'; they readily quoted examples of acquaintances or kin who had smoked Woodbine all their lives and survived to a ripe old age, while non-smoking, non-drinking contemporaries died of cancer or heart disease in their 50s.

Some of the younger generation, as might be expected, were more conscious of physical fitness. Few had the time, energy or motivation to practise health-promoting behaviour, however: some said things like 'People who play sport and games would be fitter, but we don't', as if such activities were not for 'people like us'. In general they expressed very similar ideas to the older generation:

> I'm nae een o' this health-food fanatics—this keep-fit classes. (M22)
> Well, there's one thing I dinna believe in—this efter you hae a baby in hospital, them makin' you dee a' this stupid exercises. I never did mine. I used to aye go through an' hae a smoke or somethin'.(M40)

Obesity was common in both generations, and this caused some conflict with their doctors; as one grandmother said 'When we wis a' younger, there was hundreds of folk overweight—they never went on an' on aboot it!' The young women were even more aggressive: if overweight was, as doctors said, a medical problem, then medical means should be available for dealing with it. Some had, indeed, obtained slimming drugs from their doctor, but they insisted that appearance, rather than health, was their primary concern.

Attitudes to Illness

Health, to these women, was thus either the absence of the symptoms of illness, or the refusal to admit their existence, the ability to define illnesses as normal, or the determination to 'carry on' despite illness. In a manner reminiscent of the respondents of Koos[11] in America in the 1950s, those of the older women who had raised families in particularly difficult circumstances claimed that they had no *time* to be ill themselves:

> If I was ill I still had to get up and work, you couldn't be ill—of course, the war, you didn't have time to worry about illnesses. (G17)

and they admitted that the illness of children might equally have been ignored if other problems were more salient:

> Because I was a widow for eight years, I hadn't time to mollycoddle them and run to the hospital or doctors—I was out working, I had my house, I had them. (G22, who described her children as 'healthy' despite a very bad record)

Another important factor, given the circumstances in which they brought up their families, was their conception of 'normal' illnesses, especially amongst children—troubles which were or are common, the type of things that 'people like us' could expect to suffer in large families, especially before the days of medical advance. There was also a tendency among the grandmothers to normalise some of their chronic conditions, i.e. to dismiss them as illness since they had become so used to their presence. In a similar way the women might continue to present themselves as healthy if they considered their conditions to be an inevitable consequence of being a woman, or of growing old. The illnesses might then come to be seen as normal and to be accepted. For example, many women accepted what G1 described as 'the trials of pregnancy'; another woman said, although her blood pressure was extremely high in the latter stages of pregnancy and she was admitted to hospital for some time before her son was born:

> B., again no bother with him—I had a lot of sickness during pregnancy, from the start to the finish, but otherwise I was very healthy during pregnancy.(G29)

Similarly, most of them *expected* to get hot flushes and 'women's troubles' at their time of life—'That's just nature.' To a certain extent this view was reported as being reinforced by the medical profession. In many cases this led to delay in seeking help or refusing to take any medication offered:

> But me, I've come through a' [all] I've come through—it's only me I'm hurtin' now . . . an' if I got anither pain I wid just tak' it—it wis the menopause again.(G19)

Although most of this generation were of menopausal age, comparatively few had defined their symptoms as an illness (Table 3.2).

Similarly, many of the grandmothers believed that a certain amount of 'wear and tear over the years' was inevitable. For instance, G9, aged 47, who defined herself as a healthy person, had suffered from a painful and swollen leg since she broke it five years previously and she assumed that 'arthritis had set in'. She tended to view the condition as chronic, not only because her general practitioner had led her to believe that nothing more could be done, but also because of her *age*: 'I'm gettin' on in years so I'm nae really bothered now' and G38, aged 47, similarly attributed her dizziness to advancing years:

> 'Cos as you get older, you just sorta say, that's that—just age problems, and I just thought well, it would be that, and so just let it slide by.

It seemed that the accelerated life patterns of this generation, with early childbearing and young grandmotherhood, and for many early widowhood, had resulted in a notable acceptance of ageing and deterioration as compatible with normal health.

Their daughters similarly talked as though they were older than their years. For instance, one young mother of 24 said, talking of breast-feeding:

At first you think about your figure. But it doesn't matter so much with your third if your breasts stretch a little, by that time your figure is pretty far gone anyway.(M8)

These young women, like their mothers, could reconcile illness with good health if the problems were seen as normal for 'people like us', common in their class, area or age-group, or a natural stage which any person or child could expect to pass through. Many of their children's troubles were non-illnesses which did not 'count'. This discussion of the young mothers' definitions of illness will be amplified in chapter 6.

Illness as a Moral Category

For these women—as for most people, of course—'health' was a good quality to lay claim to, and few would wish to describe themselves as anything but healthy if it were at all possible to sustain the definition with any credibility. Even more, they would not wish to say that their families were unhealthy, for this might reflect on their mothering competence. It has to be taken into account that this analysis is of the women's *presentations*, and there may have been deliberate and understandable attempts to offer a picture which minimised illness. On the other hand, the equally understandable and common liking for talking about illness, especially among the older generation, ran counter to any tendency of this sort. Also, the length of the interviews and the longitudinal nature of the association with the young families made any deliberate presentation difficult to maintain with consistency. We believe that examination of each data set as a whole, bearing in mind the possibility of conventional and not very meaningful replies to early questions, did demonstrate that illness was an important moral category; what was being expressed was a very salient attitude.

It has often been noted, of course, that the concept of illness has moral connotations.[12] Erde,[9] for instance, pointed out that disease language is infused 'with symbolic meaningfulness, mystery and dread, for example as punitive for or expressive of weakness, sin, evil or immorality', and noted that 'economic metaphors (wasting away, and rapid cell growth) and military metaphors (invasion, and under attack) will lead patients and doctors alike to conceive of a condition in moral terms'.

A constant theme of our respondents' talk was the conception of illness as a state of spiritual or moral, rather than physical, malaise. Illness (particularly in other people rather than oneself, of course) was a lack of moral fibre, a product of the imagination. Interestingly, several women of each generation associated the ideas of 'illness' and 'unhappiness', or 'health' (defined as absence of illness) and 'happiness'. Trying to explain in what way they felt ill, they said 'I'm just not happy', or accounting for freedom from illness, they said 'A happy personality helps' or 'It has a lot to do with being happy':

> I just think if you dee a normal day's work an' just eat an' be relaxed, try an' be happy within yoursel', nae ging [go] aboot moanin' an' groanin'—I think it's up to yoursel', your outlook on life.(G31)

People were not ill if they did not 'lie down to it', 'dwell on it', or 'let it get them down'. Illness was not so much the experience of symptoms, as the reaction to symptoms: the adoption of the role of a sick person by staying off work, taking to bed, or allowing one's functioning to be disturbed. 'If you're the moaning kind', they said, 'you'll aye find trouble.'

This sturdy moral view was perhaps expressed most consistently by the older generation. They believed strongly in 'mind over matter':

> I think if you brood too much on your bitties and piecies, I think you would be ill, you would. Self-analysis every morning—tell yourself, get a move on! Dinna sit an' hang aboot.(G63)

and the majority repeated again and again how much of illness was 'imagination', 'hypochondria', or 'self-indulgence', or could be overcome by strength of character:

> Sometimes—well, you can imagine a lot o' illnesses, ken. I ken mysel', if I've got a sair heid and my husband says, 'Fit's a'dee wi' you?', 'I've got a sair heid.' He'll say, 'Well, awa' to your bed'—I'll be creepin' up the stair, ken, an' lie doon, an' I'll feel sorry for myself. But if he says to me, 'Oh, there's aye somethin' a'dee wi' you', ken,—fair enough, I'll wash the dishes and away, ken.(G30)

Sometimes the grandmothers explicitly associated these attitudes with the difficult circumstances of their early lives. Their daughters often expressed similar views, however:

I've never been ill. I hate being ill. I canna stand illness. Ken? I
canna be deein' wi' it. I think it's ridiculous. With the result that if
I'm nae weel, I think, ugh, don't be stupid, I'm nae really ill.(M5)

Several others said that people 'like to think they are ill', or a lot of
illness is 'psychological'. These views were not usually applied to
young children, who were not believed to have the capacity or desire
to dramatise or malinger. Yet as the children grew older, their
mothers began increasingly to judge them by their own standards.
Rather more notably for girls than for boys, complaints of
symptoms might be described as 'moaning and groaning', 'acting
up', or 'just playing on it'.

If, in the face of this moral view, the experience of ill health is
inescapable—and for the older generation, in particular, it
was—then the obvious refuge is in fatalism. Thus, for a proportion
of the women, if they were not to judge others harshly or accept
blame themselves, 'bad luck' was the concept they had to fall back
on:

If an illness is there, it's there, ken? And you can either see about
it or forget about it. It's up to youself what you dae.(M5)

Minor illness could be ignored, and chronic complaints defined as
normal if they did not prevent ordinary functioning. More serious
disease was simply luck:

Thinks like caulds and a'thing like that I dinna think means onything because a'body gets things like that. It's just big illnesses,
they canna be helped, they're there, and they winna go
away . . . (M36)

These views obviously had important implications for the women's
attitudes to, and use of, medical services.

Concepts of Disease

It is obvious, from the preceding discussion, that this group of
women distinguished the concepts of 'illness' and 'disease' very
clearly. It was possible to have a disease without being ill, and mandatory to reject the role of sickness as far as possible even in the
presence of disease. Disease and health could, to a certain extent, co-
exist: 'Diabetes is over and above health . . . I've good health for a
diabetic.'(M39)

The rejection of illness did not, however, mean that disease was a
subject of little interest, especially for the older generation. They
talked of it at length. It can be suggested, however, that diseases as
specific entities have two dimensions by which they attach to the lives

of those who suffer them—cause, the explanatory dimension, and prognosis, the forecasting dimension. It was conspicuously the first that the women spoke of more.

There was a group of 'dreaded' diseases where, obviously, it was the prognosis that they feared. Several grandmothers spoke of their parents or themselves living in fear of tuberculosis or polio, because they were thought to be incurable or to leave the sufferer disabled. At the present time the serious diseases were those seen as the modern 'killers'—cancer, leukaemia, cerebral haemorrhage and heart disease. There was little talk, however, about the possible outcomes of any diseases at present suffered by the women or their families. They were not optimistic about cures, but both younger and older women seemed relatively incurious about the exact treatment they had received, or about the prognosis for the future. On the other hand, there was a great deal of talk about causes.

It has, of course, frequently been pointed out before that it is normal and natural for the individual to strive to provide explanations for bodily states, using whatever evidence is available to him. As Bury and Wood have commented:

Suffering without explanation is particularly hard to bear. Thus the disturbing reality of disease experience gives rise to questions—Why me? and Why now? The offering of a diagnosis or label is not enough and anxiety will be alleviated only if some indication is given of how the situation might have come about.[13]

Throughout the interviews it was obvious that for these women the most frightening symptoms were those for which no explanation could be produced, and it was these for which help was sought most readily. Again, there is an echo of the respondent of Koos[11] who said:

If I had a bad backache for two weeks, like that list says, I think I'd go to a doctor, but I can't say for sure. If I knew how I did it—say from lifting a bucket of coal—I might not go as quick as if I didn't know where it came from.

A detailed linguistic analysis of a proportion of the interview transcripts demonstrated what categories of etiology the women used, and which diseases they tended to use them for. Many of these lay notions of cause were, of course, factually wrong, and opinions about specific diseases differed widely. Certain categories were, however, much more popular than others. Infective and environmental factors—climate, damp, harmful agents or surroundings at work—were very popular causes, especially for chest conditions. The older women were also very ready to ascribe disease to stress and neglect:

> ...three times in the city hospital with tuberculosis—I called it neglect. Well, I had pleurisy before my twins were born, and I cracked my ribs just before A. was born. And I took pleurisy, and I had naebody in, wi' six o' them, you know. And I had pleurisy, and there wis naebody to look efter me, I just used to come an' get my poultice and heat it at the fire and put it back on. I ken whit it wis, it wis really neglect, my own—well, no' my own fault, I had to look efter my bairns, you understand.(G7)

Heredity was given much more weight than medical science might give it, especially by the older generation: almost every common disease was described, with a great deal of involved detail, as being 'in the family' by at least one of the respondents. Since many conditions had in fact repeated themselves through several generations of a poor environment, their reasoning was not illogical, and the appeal to heredity appeared to provide a justification for fatalism:

> Well, my sister had epilepsy, and my brother-in-law. In fact, my husband used to take them when he was little, I just found that oot nae long ago frae his mother. So fit do you expect—if it's in the family it's going to happen.(M2)

On the other hand, the women were much less ready than medical science might be to accept as causes normal degeneration, the wearing out of bodily systems, simple physiological accident, the unknown or the idiopathic. Although to a certain extent their theories were inevitably shaped by the popular media and interaction with the medical profession, the influence of their life histories on the older women was perhaps more important. Hence the emphasis on infectious disease and the preference for environmental, climatic and 'neglect' explanations. It was perhaps also less frightening to blame the environment, or even one's own behaviour, than to accept that one's body simply 'went wrong'.

The younger generation were a little less likely than the older to expand upon the cause of disease, and more likely to say 'I never thought why I had it' or to speak of diseases as 'just happening'. More of them also seemed to be basing their theories of causation upon what they had been told by the medical profession. They did not, of course, as their mothers did, have the fruits of long experience and pondering on family health to offer. 'Neglect' explanations were understandably less popular with the younger women:

> At one time it would have been lack of food and lack of vitamins. Not so much now. There's nobody starving now.(M22)

For similar reasons, they stressed a poor environment rather less, but heredity, stress, and individual susceptibility continued to be popular, as did 'natural process' explanations. Indeed, theories of causation involving pregnancy and childbirth appeared to be more widespread among the younger generation, no doubt because of their closer proximity to the actual events. Several of the young women said 'I was never right since I had family' or 'A woman is never the same after she has family.' Similarly, the young women mentioned perinatal factors as the cause of illness in their children, or, for both themselves and their children, and to a much greater extent than their mothers, the side effects of medical procedures or medication. For themselves, they stressed particularly the effects of oral contraceptives.

Overall, however, the most notable impression was of the complexity and subtlety of the thinking of both generations about the etiology of disease. They made very strenuous efforts to see their health histories as connected wholes: it was not reasonable to them that one of their bodily systems might go wrong this year, and another the next, in totally disconnected fashion. Thus there was a strain towards connecting different episodes causally. A sophisticated view of chains of cause, of immune systems, and of genetically influenced susceptibility was demonstrated. The women were also very conscious of a mind/body link. In short, though their facts may have been wrong, their basic models were no different from those of advanced medical science. One woman explained, for instance, that ulcers *must* be hereditary, since all the children 'took' them from their father, even those who lived in America, so there could be no dietary cause. Another sought to understand why diseases which she did not think were hereditary did seem to run through families:

> You know, you've got the informations in your body about diseases and how to fight them. I think that might be sort of inherited . . . of course, if low resistance runs in a family it would *look* as though all those diseases run in a family, because if you've got low resistance you're going to catch everything that's going about. That might be what it is.(M8)

The lively and independent way in which a high proportion of these minimally educated women spoke about the causes of ill health may, finally, be illustrated by one extended quotation:

> When I wis bringin' up my kids, I was forever in at the doctor and I had like a chemist shop—I had tablets to mak' me sleep, I had tablets for heidaches, an' tablets for stomach aches, an' I just said

tae mysel', tablets, tablets—I ta'en them a' an' I pit them in the bucket. I says, now they're nae helpin' me, I've got tae dae it mysel'. So I got to work an' worked things oot mysel' . . . When I first got that heidaches, I thought I was goin' aff the heid. They put me to the [psychiatric hospital]. He [husband] says, 'You're a nut.' I says, 'Well, I'll be a nut, but I'll find out I am a nut, I'll ging to a psychiatrist.' A' they asked about was sex—well, it had nuthin' a'dee wi' sex. An' then it dawned on me fit it wis—the strain o' the kids were gettin' ower much for me an' I wis against him [husband] for aye bein' awa'! See? An' then, when things would crack up, I'd maybe smack them, for maybe little. I would sit doon an' greet—I shouldn't have hutten them. Ken? An' the heidaches would get worse an' worse—an' worse . . . Ken, gettin' tae ken things, has a lot to dee wi' it—ignorance is a lot tae dee wi' bad health.(G19)

Attitudes to Medicine

The way in which these beliefs and attitudes were expressed in action, in the treatment of illness and the use made of medical services, was affected of course by another set of attitudes—ideas about medicine, its efficacy and efficiency, and about the proper use of doctors. Discussion of these is reserved for a later chapter. Between, we present the factual data concerning the health of the children and the health-related behaviour of the 58 families.

References

[1] Field, D. (1976), 'The social definition of illness' in Tuckett, D. (ed.), *An Introduction to Medical Sociology*, London: Tavistock.

[2] Fabrega, H. (1975), 'The need for an ethnomedical science', *Science*, **189**, 969.

[3] Eisenberg, L. (1977), 'Diseases and illness: distinctions between professional and popular ideas of sickness', *Culture, Medicine and Psychiatry*, **1**, 9.

[4] Tillich, P. (1961), 'The meaning of health', *Persp. Biol. and Med.*, **5**, 92.

[5] Jago, J. D. (1975), ' "Hal"—old word, new task', *Soc. Sci. and Med.*, **9**, 1.

[6] Twaddle, A. C. (1974), 'The concept of health status', *Soc. Sci. and Med.*, **8**, 29.

[7] Berg, O. (1975), 'Health and quality of life', *Acta Sociologia*, **18**, 1.

[8] Herzlich, C. (1973), *Health and Illness: A Social Psychological Analysis*, London: Academic Press.

[9] Erde, E. L. (1979), 'Philosophical considerations regarding defining "health", "disease", etc. and their bearing on medical practice', *Ethics in Sci. and Med.*, **6**, 31.

[10] Blaxter, M. (1976), *The Meaning of Disability*, London: Heinemann Educational Books.

[11] Koos, E. L. (1954), *The Health of Regionsville: What the People Thought and Did about It*, New York: Columbia University Press.

[12] e.g. Sontag, S. (1979), *Illness as Metaphor*, London: Allan Lane.

[13] Bury, M. R. and Wood, P. H. N. (1979), 'Problems of communication in chronic illness', *Internat. Rehab. Med.*, **1**, 130.

5 The Children: Illness Episodes and Health-Service Use over Six Months

We now turn to the health of the third generation. During the six-months' survey period, the young mothers reported to us 895 episodes of illness for the 139 children. For these illnesses, there were 488 consultations with doctors or other professionals within the Health Service.

The definition of an 'illness episode' remains, of course, with the mothers. There is no way in which we can compare the objective seriousness of, for instance, the respiratory infection which one mother might report as an illness, with the similar symptoms which another might not think worth mentioning. The method of questioning attempted to ensure as much consistency as possible in reporting, but of course there may have been mothers who frequently failed to notice symptoms in their children, forgot episodes which had occurred, or deliberately did not tell us about them. Because of the nature of the prompting—'Have they had any colds? any stomach upsets?'—many trivial symptoms are included which the mothers might not otherwise have defined as 'proper illnesses'.

The attitudes to health and sickness which have been described obviously affect what is to count as illness—illness to be reported in the survey, as well as illness to be treated or taken for professional help. The way in which these symptoms were recognised and given meaning is discussed in chapter 6; here, it may simply be noted that, as shown in Table 5.1, the mother reported an average of about one illness episode a month per child. Slightly more illnesses were reported for boys than for girls.

Table 5.1   Illness episodes reported per child during six months

	Male	Female	All children
Mean number of episodes	7.14	5.74	6.44
(Number of children)	(69)	(70)	(139)

For the purpose of this analysis, 'episodes' include not only acute illnesses, or accidents, but also chronic conditions which the mother mentioned as being troublesome during that month. Dental decay is also included if it was mentioned by the mother.

To think in terms of averages is perhaps misleading, since as might be expected the range was very great—from no episodes at all during the six months to a maximum of 25. In any family there might, of course, be one particular child, perhaps suffering from several chronic conditions, with a large number of reported illness episodes. An examination of the family patterns of reporting, however, showed that—these special children apart—there was a marked likelihood of high, or low, reporting for all the children of the family. In some families, few illnesses would be reported for any child, and in others there would be many for each of the children. Obviously there is no way of determining, on this evidence alone, whether the health of the children in high-reporting families was 'worse' in any objective way, or whether these mothers were simply more meticulous in noting, remembering, or reporting symptoms. The relationship between various indicators of actual health and the mothers' health behaviour will be considered in subsequent chapters.

One slight but regular trend in reporting was for the average number of illnesses per child to become less as family size increased (see Table 5.2). It is sometimes suggested that there is more ill health in large families, because of the spread of infection and because of possible association with a poorer environment. Since most of our families have two or three children the numbers are small in other groups, but it does seem here that the mothers of smaller families, perhaps having more time for each child, were likely to report more illness episodes.

Table 5.2 Relationship of family size to the reporting of illness episodes

	Family size			
	1 child	2 children	3 children	4 children
Mean episodes per child	7.8	6.5	6.1	5.7
(Number of families)	(5)	(29)	(20)	(4)

An analysis was also made of the patterns of reporting according to the time of year. (Because the survey was spread over parts of two calendar years, it was not possible for the survey months to be exactly similar in every family, but for the majority some winter or early spring months were included.) The expected distribution emerged. More acute episodes—largely respiratory infections—were reported in winter, and the number of children who were troubled by chronic conditions was also greater in the winter months. There was a high incidence of infectious diseases in the spring of one year. Accidents, on the other hand, appeared to be unrelated to the season of the year, and about one child in ten was reported to have had an accident in any given month.

There are really no comparable data by which these rates of perceived illness in children can be judged to be greater, or less, than those found in families in other social groups or geographical areas. Surveys of the prevalence of symptoms in adults[1] have often found much higher rates of illness, but they are usually based on responses to a checklist of symptoms, rather than requests for 'illnesses' as defined by the respondent herself. The figures presented in the General Household Survey (GHS)—which are similarly based on mothers' reports—may have some limited relevance, although information about children has been restricted in recent volumes.[2] In 1976, 'acute illness', defined as illness which 'restricted normal activity' was recorded at rates, in Scotland, which represent an average of about eight days acute illness per child per year. Obviously, this is less than our families' average of 13 illness episodes per child per year, though the GHS criterion of 'restricted activity' may of course be problematic in a child. It may be noted, however, that the GHS has consistently found, as in our own families, that less illness is reported for girls than for boys.

Consultations
There is better justification for a quantified description of the consultations during the survey period. It is less likely that mothers forgot or omitted to report visits to the doctor or other services, nor is it likely that they pretended to use services when they had not, since they knew they would be asked for accounts of what was said or done. We therefore believe that we have an unusually full and accurate record of all the use of health services for the 139 children over six months.

'Consultations' are here being defined solely as consultations with health-service personnel, reserving for a later chapter discussion of advice-seeking from family, friends or pharmacists. They include surgery consultations with a general practitioner, home visits by the practitioner, attendance at the accident and emergency department of the hospital or at outpatient clinics, admission to hospital as an inpatient, treatment by a dentist, and consultations or treatment at specialist clinics such as speech therapy, audiology, or educational psychology. Visits to child health clinics (where a doctor or a health visitor might be consulted) are also included, and patient-initiated contacts with health visitors, in cases where the mother was seeking a consultation about a specific problem. Routine visits of the mothers to clinics for baby weighing, assessment and immunisation are not included, nor health visitor-initiated visits to the family. 'Joint' consultations, where more than one child was taken to the doctor at the same time, or the doctor visited two children who were ill, have been counted as a consultation for each child involved.

Table 5.3 Consultations with health services during six months

	Males Age 0–4	Males Age 5–12	Females Age 0–4	Females Age 5–12	All children
Average number of consultations per child during six months	3.08	4.60	3.55	2.97	3.51
(Number of children)	(39)	(30)	(38)	(32)	(139)

As Table 5.3 shows, the children were referred to health services roughly once every six weeks; for every three illness episodes reported there were about two consultations. Table 5.4 shows which services these consultations were with, expressed as rates per year for

Table 5.4 Rates of consultation, child per year

Consultations with:	Male	Female	All children aged 0–12	All children aged 5–12	All children
General practitioner	3.74	4.80	4.83	3.58	4.27
At surgery	2.15	2.81	2.78	2.10	2.47
By telephone	0.17	0.22	0.26	0.13	0.20
Home visit	1.42	1.77	1.79	1.35	1.60
Clinic doctor or health visitor (patient-initiated; not routine)	0.49	0.17	0.44	0.19	0.33
Hospital Accident and emergency department	0.35	0.46	0.26	0.58	0.40
Outpatient clinic	1.13	0.28	0.62	0.79	0.70
Admission as inpatient	0.26	0.17	0.21	0.23	0.22
Dentist	1.04	0.51	0.18	1.52	0.78
Other specialist service	0.41	0.23	0.13	0.56	0.32
(Number of children)	(69)	(70)	(77)	(62)	(139)

easier comparison with other data. (There should be a record of 139 × 6 'child-months', 834, but 10 arc missing for various reasons such as mother in hospital, new baby born during six months, etc. In every case where rates are quoted, allowance has been made for these 'missing' months.)

In summary, consultations with a general practitioner were made for these children at a rate of about 4 per year, and they had about 1.5 contacts per year with the hospital. Children over 5 had an average of about 1.5 contacts with a dentist per year. There was some use of clinic doctors or health visitors for consultations about specific symptoms or illnesses, and this was not necessarily confined to children under school age.

The rates of consultation with general practitioners may be compared with those reported in the Second National Study (1970–71) of morbidity in general practice.[3] These are, of course, for England and Wales. Children under 5 were reported as having an average of 3.8 (males) and 3.5 (females) consultations with a GP per year, and older children 1.9 (both sexes). In the General Household Survey, 1977, children under 5 in Scotland had 6.0 (males) and 4.0 (females) consultations per year, and older children 2.4 (males) and 1.6 (females). It may be noted that consultation rates are consistently shown as being lower (as far as older children are concerned) in Scotland than in England and Wales.

These rates are for all social classes, and it must be noted that British statistics (such as earlier editions of the GHS) have consistently shown that, for children, rates of consultation decline from social class I to social class V. This is the opposite of the adult trend, where social classes IV and V are usually shown to have the highest consulting rates. The rates in our sample appear to be higher than those usually reported for social classes IV and V, and the children certainly received a higher proportion of their general practitioner consultations at home (see Table 5.5).

Table 5.5 Site of GP consultations, General Household Survey and this sample compared

| | Per cent of consultations with GP | | |
	At surgery	At home	By telephone
GHS 1977, Great Britain			
Children 0–4	78	17	5
Children 5–14	84	10	6
This sample			
Children 0–4	57	37	6
Children 5–11	59	38	3

Rates of attendance at, or admission to, hospital are more difficult to compare. The GHS has usually suggested that, in Scotland, in all social classes, about 6–15 per cent of children are reported as having attended an outpatient department during a three-month period. The figure for boys is usually greater than that for girls, and in our sample the difference is conspicuous. The rate of nearly one visit per child per year in these children included individual children with repeated visits, but nevertheless seems high. The rates of attendance at the accident and emergency department are also high, but these are influenced by the mothers' preference (discussed later in connection with accidents) for using this service.

The sample is perhaps too small for generalisations to be made about admissions to hospital, especially as clear national statistics are lacking. The rate of one child in five per year is also high, however. Considering not simply the six-months' record, but the history of admissions to hospital of each child which the mothers described to us, only a minority of children of any age had *never* been treated in hospital. In the National Child Development Survey, the proportion 'ever admitted to hospital' at 7 years of age in social class V children was 47.3 per cent.[3] The admission rate of this sample was certainly higher than this, though it cannot be assumed that this indicates more, or more serious, illness, rather than reflecting particular referral or admission practices on the part of doctors.

Conditions for Which Professional Help Was Sought

If the mother of a child perceived that a medical consultation was necessary various alternatives were open: she could choose to present it to a general practitioner at his surgery, or call the practitioner to the home, or take the child for consultation with a doctor or health visitor at a child health clinic, or seek treatment from the accident and emergency department of the children's hospital. Table 5.6 lists the commonest medical conditions, broadly defined, which prompted these consultations, and shows how the consultations were distributed among the alternatives. Outpatient clinics and admissions to hospital are omitted, since these are not primary resources open for the mother to choose. The consultations listed under 'general practitioner—surgery' include the few which were made by telephone. Most of these concerned respiratory infections in young children, or rashes thought to be rubella.

It is obvious that the general practitioner's work, for these children, was predominantly in connection with a limited number of types of condition. Table 5.7 shows, for older and younger children, which conditions made up the greater part of the surgery 'load', and which

Table 5.6 *Where consultations were made during six months*

Condition	General practitioner		Clinic or health visitor	Accident and emergency dept	(N = 100%)
	At surgery	Home visit			
Respiratory infections	62	27	10	—	(77)
Accidents (cuts, bruises, fractures, bites, etc.)	15	—	(1)ᵃ	82	(39)
Childhood infectious diseases (measles, mumps, whooping cough, chickenpox)	18	77	(2)	—	(39)
Tonsillitis, sore throat, sinusitis	65	30	(2)	—	(37)
Gastrointestinal symptoms	48	48	(1)	—	(31)
Ear conditions	84	(2)	(2)	—	(25)
Rubella	50	50	—	—	(20)
Skin conditions, eczema, rash	67	(3)	(3)	—	(18)
Urinary infections	(6)	(1)	—	—	(7)
Mouth infections, herpes	(4)	(3)	—	—	(7)
Eye conditions	—	—	(6)	—	(6)
Enuresis	(6)	—	—	—	(6)
Convulsions, epilepsy	(2)	(3)	—	(1)	(6)
Otherᵇ	50	46	(1)	—	(28)

Notes: ᵃ actual numbers in brackets
   ᵇ includes: bronchitis, diabetes, allergies, overweight, poisoning, object up nose, breast lump, alopaecia, sunburn, circulation problems, behaviour problems, nightmares, burns, scalds, orthopaedic problems, swollen glands, general advice

Table 5.7 Consultations at the surgery compared with home visits, per cent

	Age 0–4		Age 5–12	
Condition	At surgery, clinic or by telephone	At home	At surgery, clinic or by telephone	At home
Respiratory infections	34	24	17	10
Accidents	5	—	1	—
Childhood infectious diseases (excl. rubella)	7	22	—	38
Tonsillitis, sore throat, sinusitis	8	7	22	16
Gastrointestinal symptoms	9	16	7	10
Ear conditions	6	3	21	—
Rubella	5	4	4	12
Skin conditions, eczema, rash	9	3	4	2
Urinary infections	4	1	1	—
Enuresis	—	—	8	—
Mouth infections, herpes	1	4	4	—
Other	12	16	11	—
(N = 100%)	(134)	(68)	(75)	(42)

made up the general practitioner's home visits. For pre-school children, respiratory infections (many of them, of course, in quite young infants) and infectious diseases were the most common causes of the doctor's being called out, although it may be noted that several cases of infectious disease were taken to the surgery or clinic. For school-age children, calls to the home were predominantly for whooping cough and measles, though there was also a high proportion for infections diagnosed as rubella. In the surgery, throat and ear symptoms were the ones most commonly presented for these older children.

Rates of Consultation and 'Disadvantage'
The families may be divided into 'high consulting' and 'low consulting' groups according to the average number of consultations (of all sorts) made, during the six months, per child in the family. There were 35 families whose consultations numbered less than the average 3.5, and 23 families whose averages were higher. Without relating these to the actual health of the children, no conclusions can be drawn, of course, about the mothers' relative readiness to consult. It was noted (p.   ) that the families were divided into two groups according to a composite index of disadvantage, however,

and it does seem of interest to ask whether it was the 'more' or the 'less' disadvantaged who were likely to be high, or low, consulters.

Table 5.8   Index of disadvantage and number of consultations

Families whose number of consultations per child was:	Families categorised as	
	'More' disadvantaged	'Less' disadvantaged
Below average	21	14
Above average	8	15
(Number of families)	(29)	(29)

Table 5.8 shows that while the 'less' socially disadvantaged amongst these families could be either high or low consulters, there seemed to be some likelihood of the 'more' disadvantaged consulting less frequently than the average. A significant part of this difference was caused by a lesser likelihood of consultations with a dentist, rather than a doctor. Nevertheless the possibility that some of those in the poorest circumstances may be less likely either to perceive symptoms in their children as illness, or to consult about them, is one preliminary finding that must be borne in mind in the considerations of the children's health and the mothers' health-care behaviour which follow.

References
[1] e.g. Wadsworth, M. E. J., Butterfield, W. J. H. and Blaney, R. (1971), *Health and Sickness: the Choice of Treatment*, London: Tavistock.
Banks, M. H., Beresford, S. A. A., Morrell, D. C., Waller, J. J. and Watkins, C. J. (1978), 'Symptom recording and demand for primary medical care in women aged twenty to forty-four years' in Tuckett, D. (ed.), *Basic Readings in Medical Sociology*, London: Tavistock.

[2] *General Household Survey* (1976), London: HMSO.

[3] Davie, R., Butler, N. and Goldstein, H. (1972), *From Birth to Seven: the Second Report of the National Child Development Study (1958 Cohort)*, London: Longman.

6 The Children: the Mothers' Perception of Symptoms

How did the mothers (and sometimes the grandmothers) interpret the signs and symptoms which went to make up the record of illness episodes during six months which has been described? In this chapter we present a descriptive account based on an examination of the womens' report of each episode, together with more general comments which they made in discussion.

It has, of course, frequently been noted in studies of 'illness behaviour' that perceptions of the meaning of particular symptoms are socially differentiated. Ethnic origin,[1] age[2] and social class[3] are three of the variables which were frequently shown, in early American studies, to affect the way in which a symptom is defined as 'ill' or 'not ill'. In particular, evidence has suggested that people in poorer social circumstances may have higher thresholds of tolerance for symptoms which are not functionally incapacitating, or are seen as normal in the context of their life situations; as Mechanic[4] said:

> People who work long hours expect to be tired, and are therefore less likely to see tiredness as indicative of an illness. Persons who do heavy physical work are more likely to attribute such symptoms as backache to the nature of their lives and work rather than to an illness condition.

The analysis here is of course of the perception of symptoms in *children*, and there is little knowledge about any systematic difference between different groups of mothers in the meaning that they give to their children's symptoms. The mothers belong to one particular social and regional group, and no comparison is available with other groups. It may, however, be possible to compare their definition of the meaning or the seriousness of symptoms with those which their doctors appeared to be applying, and to consider the implications for the families' use of services.

It must be noted as a preliminary point that, despite the fact that this sample shared a similar social background, environment, and education, no principles for the interpretation of specific symptoms could be found which applied universally. Similar conditions might elicit entirely different responses in different women. In general, the events of the six-months' survey, while often supporting and supplementing previous findings, demonstrate primarily the complexities of 'illness behaviour' and the limitations of simple models.

Reported Symptoms

The list of signs and behaviours which were related in response to questioning is of course extensive; these were the 'triggers' which initiated feelings that something was not quite as it should be, although they were not invariably defined as 'illness'. Some symptoms were 'obvious' and common, others less so; frequently appearing in combinations, they might be noticed first when the child complained. The mother herself may have perceived the change, or it may have been a relative, friend or teacher.

The symptoms were described in a variety of ways, related to how they impinged on the mother:

(1) *Heard*: these were complaints of pain or unpleasant sensation, general or in a particular site (head, eyes, mouth, throat, stomach, etc.) or at certain times (e.g. when passing water), in the form of 'screaming', 'crying', girning', 'sobbing', 'whining', 'moaning', 'pinging', depending on the age of the child; if not voiced, complaint may be indicated by rubbing or scratching the affected part. Other relevant noises were coughing ('croupy', 'dry', 'sore', 'bark'), 'wheezing', 'sneezing', 'sniffling', 'snochering', 'gasping', 'choking', 'cowking' (retching), 'hoarse'/'thick'/'froggy' speech, lisping, stuttering, mispronunciation, 'talking baby'.

(2) *Felt*: changes of body temperature described as 'hot', 'sweating', 'fevered', 'cold to touch', 'shivery'; perhaps swelling and lumps.

(3) *Smelt*: e.g. 'bad breath' and 'smelly' nasal discharge.

(4) *Seen*: (a) changes in bodily state, e.g. colour—'pale', 'white', 'red', 'flushed', 'blue', 'almost black'—in various parts of the body, particularly the face; shape and texture of the skin—'spots', 'rashes', 'dry skin', 'scaley', 'blisters', 'sores', 'sties', 'boils', 'abscesses', 'puffiness', swelling and lumps, extreme slimness or loss of weight, and rapid weight gain.
(b) 'unnatural' fluids and discharges, e.g. blood, pus, etc. from ears, eyes, nose, mouth, front and back passages, described, for instance, as 'weepy eyes', 'sticky eyes', 'slivering', 'streaming cold', 'blood in the nappy'; vomiting ('natural' in babies but not when 'like a

spout'); more or less frequent bowel movements or passing water, change in appearance or texture of stools and urine; loss of control over bladder or bowels after this had been established, or 'late' control (depending on the mother's norms).

(c) unconsciousness or 'black-outs', loss of movement in part of the body such as an arm or leg, 'limpness', 'weak', the state of being 'away', 'starey', 'looking funny—he didn't seem to know us', and 'classic' signs of convulsion such as rolling eyes and jerking limbs.

(5) *Behaviour* that was seen as strange or annoying for the mother, often consisting of less tangible signs: 'He would never look you in the eye, he would look straight through you' (M41); 'She holds her head on one side in a funny way.' (M61) Deafness was suspected when the child consistently turned up the volume on the television or did not answer when spoken to, and sight was queried when a child failed to notice Lego pieces on the floor. Children were described as 'hyperactive' and 'high', 'restless' or 'wakeful', e.g. children aged two and three would not go to bed before their parents, a three year old was awake from 4 a.m. when his postman father left home for work, a boy of $2\frac{1}{2}$ wandered around in the middle of the night, children had nightmares and fear of going to sleep alone.

A group of indicators was almost universally believed to 'mean trouble' in all the children, e.g. sleepiness, 'taking to bed', easily tired, 'lying about', being quieter than usual, or lack of appetite, especially for favourite foods. These sorts of indicators were often particularised, and the following are examples of very many similar statements:

C. started falling asleep in the afternoons and being very good—not her usual self.(M8)
I know when F. and S. are going to be unwell. They sort of hang about and their eyes go pink.(M2)
When S. refuses a biscuit I know right away there's something not right with him. Same with F. and ice-cream.(M12)

Most of the women would claim some privileged knowledge of the child's physical and emotional state, because of their special relationship; as they said, 'a mother knows', 'you know when your child's not right', 'it's instincts', 'If I thought it wasn't normal ... I think your common sense tells you.'

The Interpretation of Symptoms
Having realised that something was afoot, that the child's bodily,

mental or emotional state had changed, the mothers had to determine the significance of what was occurring, to make a preliminary decision of ill or not ill, worthy of note or of little consequence.

Certain symptoms may appear so frightening that panic and immediate action result. However, there is generally time for pondering on causation or prognosis, and other parts of the child's body may be examined; if the neck is sore, is it also swollen? if the face is swollen are there also spots? what types of spots are they—infection, infestation, or allergy? where is the rash situated? Over time the mothers may have learned, frequently from mother or sibs (or from doctors) the classic symptoms of various infectious diseases; two mothers specifically mentioned, for instance, 'spots behind the ear'. An impression of 'what's going around' may help to firm up the diagnosis about rashes, swellings, and sore throats.

A preliminary diagnosis is therefore sometimes, although not invariably, possible. Nevertheless mothers must, in the nature of things, using the information at hand and their experience and knowledge, decide or drift towards taking the symptoms or signs seriously and worthy of action. They may emphasise them and worry about them, or play them down and ignore them, biding their time. The variables affecting interpretation will be dealt with under the following headings:

(1) The intrinsically 'frightening' or 'trivial' nature of the symptoms
(2) Sites of symptoms
(3) Other intrinsic features of the symptom or the occasion
(4) The nature of 'infection'
(5) The child's health history
(6) Knowledge of causes, diagnosis and cure
(7) Practical contingencies

The intrinsically 'frightening' or 'trivial' nature of the symptoms
There were certain signs which were universally feared and known to be dangerous, for which emergency action—the calling of an ambulance, the summoning of a GP or an immediate visit to him—was likely to be taken. Some of these were 'fits', screaming, paralysis, lumps, choking, or the 'drawback' in whooping cough: symptoms which are intrinsically worrying or upsetting, or taken to indicate serious diseases. One grandmother vividly described some of these rules for immediate action:

[What sorts of things would you get the doctor for?] Well, swellin' an' things like that . . . Ken? Things like, if their throat wis badly swollen or—you could see that they were really ill, really burnin' up, their eyes bright an'—really bright—now, when a kiddy's like that I think he's really ill. When the eyes is like—there wis candles in the back o' them, sorta thing, ken. I find that's when a kiddy's really ill—their temperature really *is* high, ken. Really feverish. An' you niver know—an' ony kind o' abdominal pains or onythin' like that. To me, that is an emergency, a doctor should come in right away for that. Ken. As soon as you describe that symptoms—that doctor should be on that doorstep sorta thing, ken. Cos I mean—abdominal pain, a kiddy canna really tell you. Ken? Though they're maybe sayin' 'Sair, sair' [sore] you dinna ken—actually far [where] the sair is, ken? But nine times oot o' ten they pit their hand to the pain. Ken? Which is an automatic reaction to a grown-up, never mind to a . . . but you'll find that little eens [ones] dee it, pit their hand to the pain, ken—Cos you've a good idea far the pain is, ken. But to me, onything like that—there should be nae messin' aboot—get the doctor in right away.(G40)

During the survey months the young mothers did indeed react urgently to severe pain, convulsions, and lumps and swellings. Many mothers admitted that they always panicked at the sight of blood. Extreme distress was also caused by the symptoms ('run down', 'thin and losing weight', 'all his glands swelled up') which were believed to indicate TB.

High fever was certainly *claimed* by most of the mothers to be a worrying sign. One claimed that she always used a thermometer when she suspected a child to be running a temperature:

I don't like them running a temperature . . . it's scarey if they're not properly *with* you. It can damage their brains if it gets too high. (M61, who added that she would always check the children's temperature if a fever was suspected)

But few had thermometers and reports of action did not always back up this assertion, except for those children prone to febrile convulsions. However, temperature was often a trigger to some action when another symptom might be neglected, or it might lead to calling in the GP rather than going to the surgery. Generally the limits of 'serious' fever were set quite high; one mother said she worried if a child's temperature reached 104, and another called in the doctor when her three year old had a temperature of 103. The worrying degree of fever was 'difficult to explain—you sort of know yourself—really, really fevered'.(M28)

At the other extreme, certain complaints and symptoms were seen as so trivial, common, and self-limiting that they were not believed to necessitate undue concern, or the problem was defined as not really illness. For many mothers this included runny noses, 'snivels', 'snuffles', and in some cases coughs and flu symptoms, even when three or four children were affected. 'Little trivial things like that, I wouldn't bother the doctor'; 'I think a cold comes naturally and will go away the same way—on its own'; 'It's just the common cold that everyone has just now'; 'I wouldn't get the doctor if it was just a runny nose.' But a vast array of proprietory medicines was used to alleviate the symptoms of this 'commom complaint'.

Into the same category frequently fell throat trouble—'Just a sore throat', 'I knew it was just tonsillitis'; or 'upset stomachs', 'sickness and diarrhoea', a sty: 'Sties comes and goes— that's what I've always thought'; and a poisoned finger: 'I don't think you should go to the doctor for things like that.' Earache did not always worry mothers: 'I wouldn't say they were serious things. Just run-of-the-mill sort of things. Nothing to be anxious about.' Severe and even prolonged constipation was also not felt to warrant undue concern; for four days one mother tried all manner of preparations on her seven-year-old daughter, including her own suppositories, and another sought little medical help, but continuously used medicine from the chemist for her six-months-old son's chronic constipation.

Other conditions were not believed to necessitate medical action because they were thought to be natural and normal processes, and decidedly not illness. Conspicuous among these was teething. Symptoms such as diarrhoea, earache, prolonged colds, sticky eyes, cough, sickness, sore gums, sore bottom did not cause great worry, the mothers saying such things as—'I put it down to teething'; 'he gets it when teething'; 'it's teething bronchitis'. Despite a history of pneumonia, a six-months-old baby's cough did not cause concern because teething was believed to be the cause, and even for a girl aged nine no medical advice was sought, when she became very flushed, listless, had a head cold, and very painful gums, as her problem was defined as 'A back tooth coming through...There's nothing they can do.'(M39) It was not until the problem was redefined a week later as possible tonsillitis that she was taken to the surgery.

A similar attitude was taken to dental decay and even severe tooth-ache, which seemed to be defined in a different manner to other pain. For instance, a three year old had a visible abscess near a tooth and was in considerable pain 'So I gave him a junior aspirin, it's stopped hurting now' (M55) and his two-year-old sister was given ice-cream to stop her complaining about a possible broken tooth. Another five year old had severe toothache for a week, and an abscess developed before she saw an emergency dentist. Her mother said 'That's not important. That's not really health.' (M16)

Sites of symptoms

The involvement of certain sites in the body, most commonly 'the chest' or lungs, gave importance to symptoms for many mothers. There was symbolic significance in a cold being 'in the chest' or in 'difficulty breathing', as opposed to a 'normal cold'. One grand-mother said:

> We aye keep a check on the chests, ken—when they hae coughs, ken, to see it disnae go into their chests. We fairly check on that.(G28)

Similarly, mothers explained why they had consulted a doctor in terms such as:

> 'I was afraid of it going down to his chest' (M51); 'I always like to make sure the chest is clear' (M68); 'The only time I think you should get a doctor is if it goes into the chest' (M17); 'If I thought it was really chesty I would take her to the doctor' (M32); 'She was breathing like she had been running for a long time, breathing very fast' (M38); 'It was like comin' frae the soles o' her feet.'(M40)

Ear trouble was very prevalent among the children, but several of the mothers did not consult until the child actually seemed to be suffering some hearing impairment: when her five-year-old son first complained of earache, M1 persevered with her own drops until 'his hearing seemed dull' and after his operation she consistently did not consult about bleeding and suppurating. When the child's *eyes* were affected in some way, most mothers were concerned. For instance, M53 consulted when her daughter's eyes became sore, red and crusted and asserted that she would never try to treat eye prob-lems herself; M16 worried about her three-year old's cold when her 'eyes swelled up' and called medical help 'in case her eyes closed up completely'; M20 might not have bothered seeking help for German measles (she had not done so for her youngest child) had not the boy's eyes been affected—'the spots were in his eyes'.

Despite some talk about fear of appendicitis, and the view of G40 already quoted, *stomach pain* was an uncommon cause for concern. For instance, M1 passed off her small daughter's sore stomach 'for weeks' as a 'carry on', and despite some mention of worry about her son having appendicitis, M19 continued with home remedies for three days.

Despite some idea that *headaches* in children were rather unusual, they were not invariably a cause for concern. M41 said that she would not call in her GP, 'as some people do', 'if they were just complaining of a sore head'. However, other mothers did take their children to the doctor when they complained of back headaches, saying, for instance, 'I was very worried because kids don't usually take headaches.' (M39)

Some mothers were dramatically worried about *urinary infections* in girls, but concern could be variable. One mother sought help for her four-year-old daughter only when she started 'passing blood clots', although she said she would have consulted anyway if the child's pain had persisted.

Other intrinsic features of the symptom or the occasion

As has been commonly noted before, features of symptoms such as frequency, persistence and timing obviously affect the way in which they are perceived.[4] Among these mothers, symptoms of short duration were generally treated in a non-serious fashion, particularly vomiting and diarrhoea, earache and nose bleeds. If the symptom did not cause the child to complain, did not make him 'down', and left him 'going about' it tended to cause less concern. On the other hand, persistence and worsening of symptoms, and the failure of home remedies frequently (but not invariably) led to concern and consultation. When symptoms which might be defined as relatively unimportant lasted for days without improvement, the mothers felt that something more serious was present and summoned help: examples included vomiting, enuresis, or earache. For some mothers who would seldom consult about one problem a *combination* of symptoms was also a spur to action; for example cases where a child was sick *and* fevered, had diarrhoea *and* was eating badly; had sore throats *and* sore stomachs *and* vomiting; had a cough *and* sickness; had a heacache *and* was flushed *and* appeared to have swollen glands; was feverish, off his food, had vomiting and diarrhoea *and* a cough.

When a symptom occurred also affected interpretation. There was a general feeling that children with, say, chest problems, were more badly affected in winter and therefore the mother tended to worry more about such symptoms when it was cold: 'He's prone to take a chesty cold in winter . . . When winter comes he's usually to get his mixture.' (M6) Another mother generally kept her daughter away from the nursery in winter in case her cold developed into bronchitis, 'But I would put her to school with a cold in summer because I know she's not going to get chilled.' (M8) Awareness of 'what's going around', or 'in the building', also alerted some mothers: M25 actively checked for spots on her children because 'chicken-pox and

German measles are going around in the flats'.

The *child's age* was also important; there was a definite tendency to worry more and seek advice more quickly for babies' symptoms (if not necessarily for 'baby specific' symptoms such as teething) than for similar symptoms in older children within the family. As one mother commented 'When it's babies, you want to see [the doctor] *now.*' (M61)

Some women treated certain children's symptoms more lightly than others because they believed such conditions were *harmless at that age, 'normal' for that age*, or a '*stage*' they were going through; a few women made this explicit, although undoubtedly several more acted on an implicit assumption. For instance, a ten-year-old girl's headaches and sore stomachs were attributed to the onset of puberty, and medical advice was not sought and of another girl of nine, the mother said:

> She's all aches and pains as usual. I think it's her age—a phase she's going through. 'Oh, my arm's sore, oh, my leg's sore.' We usually just ignore her now.(M22)

Only rarely did mothers differentiate the symptoms of *boys and girls*, except for the specifically female conditions cited. Certainly, there was no indication that boys were expected to be 'tougher'. Rather, there was more likelihood of girls being accused of unwarranted fussing.

The nature of 'infection'

The reaction of the mothers to the symptoms of childhood infectious diseases were very varied, as the record of consultations (Table 5.7) indicated. The grandmother whose rules were quoted on p. 53 had gone on to say:

> [Are there any things you would tend to leave for a bit before seeing a doctor?] Aye—like kiddies'll come oot in rashes—they're a bit fretful—'Oh, the doctor, the doctor'. No, no, you leave that. It could be a heat rash or onything like that—but if it persists, get him. If feverishness persists, an' the spots persist a' the time, there's definitely somethin' there—that's needin' cleared up, ken. But, I mean, you'll find them phonin' for the doctor—it's maybe been a warm night, ken—specially wi' babies—young babies—they've maybe been hot or somethin' through the night, they've got a rash on their body; 'Oh my—'. Well, they could easy take them to the clinic. The clinic'll say 'Oh, it's only a heat rash—just the baby's been rather hot through the night.' There's a heap of things—I suppose you panic really. Aye, for the young lassies—oh, a rash—especially their first—'Oh, my God—' it's only a heat rash, ken. But—it's quite explainable.(G40)

As G40 understandingly explained, mothers frequently did panic and call the doctor to the house for rubella rashes. Some reported that infectious disease was the only thing for which they would call in medical help. On the other hand, others believed that infectious diseases were so common and 'known' that they could not possibly have serious implications. One mother requested one GP visit when two of her children appeared to have a fairly bad attack of measles, but she did not call again when the two year old developed the same or worse symptoms. Similarly, although her boy aged three had had quite a bad bout of measles the previous week, M19 did not summon help when her one-year-old son seemed to be similarly affected. Mumps could also be treated fairly lightly: although her four year old was 'screaming with a sore ear' and 'dozy', M28 took her to the GP clinic some distance away. Frequently children recovering from infectious diseases were allowed out to play with other children or returned to school sooner than the doctor had advised.

The child's health history
Some mothers explained that they were especially worried about the symptoms of certain children in their family, because of the children's health history, 'weakness' and other special characteristics. M3 believed her eight-year-old son suffered 'sort of asthma attacks' due to damp housing in the past and to lack of immunity; when he became 'fevered' or had a cough she worried that it 'might be in his chest' or might 'start up again', and consulted the doctor immediately. Other examples of past experience influencing present action include, among many others, M56 who said that she consulted for her two year old 'the minute he gets the cold' because 'I let it go once' and 'he got measles'; or M16 who became extremely worried if her toddler developed a cold, especially with a cough, because she had contracted whooping cough at three months: 'I tend to panic and get the doctor in right away—it might turn into something.' Another mother was concerned when she heard her six-year-old son cough or if he got 'really hot' as he had been admitted to hospital for choking the previous year:

> We usually get the doctor if there's something, especially after D.—we got a scare. If we hadn't got the doctor his throat might hae closed completely and he wouldn't have been able to breathe at all. So now we always like to be sure.(M21)

However, other chronic or frequent conditions could be treated lightly because they were normal for that child, the mothers were used to the problem and the diagnosis was known. For instance, one mother admitted that she was becoming less concerned over her son's eczema:

> Some days it's bad, others it's OK. He's had it so long that I've stopped getting in a state about it.(M7)

Mothers talked of their children's 'usual sore ears' or 'usual colds', and a runny nose might almost be accepted as a permanent state:

> There's not much you can do. I've tried mixtures but they don't work. He's just one of that kids that always have colds in winter—he was wheezy since birth anyway.(M38)

In the same way M41 was not concerned about her son's coughing: 'It's just his normal cough—It's quite usual for him to have a cough.'

Several other mothers treated a particular child's symptoms and complaints more seriously due to less specific characteristics. For instance, M1 believed that her younger son was less capable of 'fighting off' any condition which the other children developed —'bed and Disprin don't seem to help'—so she tended to take any illness which he contracted more seriously. On the other hand, the characteristics of an individual child could lead to the mother interpreting symptoms less seriously:

> She had a cold, but she fought it off herself. She had a runny nose, but she didn't need a mixture. She usually manages to fight off a cold herself.(M6)

Knowledge of causes, diagnosis and cure
Certain problems might be interpreted in a serious manner if the mother had knowledge of the serious consequences of the symptoms, not because of the child's history but from experience with another member of the family or even herself. For instance, one mother's reaction was 'Oh my God!' when her two year old started 'takin' a likin' for babies' dummies and that' and 'her eyes started rolling and she started shakin'—That's how it started with (her sister). I wouldn't like to go through that again. It's a lot of work.'(M2)

Other examples are M65, who was very concerned and persistent about her four year old's suspected deafness, despite a 'sharp' reaction from her GP at first, because she herself had had persistent ear trouble as a child and had been left slightly deaf, and M12 who was very annoyed about the time taken to diagnose and treat her daughter's poor eyesight, as she herself had a similar problem and G12 suffered a progressing 'eye disease'. M36 *expressed* concern (although her action did not totally endorse it) about her son's bed-wetting and headaches, since his father was epileptic 'and he used to do that ... There must be something happening in his head.'

On the other hand, if the outcome was 'known' and understood not to be life-threatening, symptoms might not be acted upon. In one family girls aged four and five were both 'bothered with infections down below', but the mother seldom sought medical help (as she had been advised to) and used home remedies: 'I just treats it mysel'. I know because I've got it mysel'.' (M16)

Also, less concern appeared to be engendered by conditions for which the *cause* was believed to be known, especially 'something going round' or 'something eaten'. Explanations for symptoms held to be not serious included: 'he must have got a draught' (eye infection in baby); 'worried about the dentist' (diarrhoea); the child being due to take a dancing exam the next day (sore stomach); 'late nights at her aunt's' (vomiting); 'too many sweets' (rash); 'they eat too much rubbish' (sickness and diarrhoea); 'but they eat a lot of snackery on a Saturday' (vomiting); 'eating ice lollies' ('a touch of diarrhoea'—although the trouble seemed to continue for several months); 'it was just a bug going around'; 'something going around', and—'a bug going around the school' (diarrhoea); 'well, it's just a virus, isn't it?' (herpes).

Practical contingencies
The way in which a range of practical factors was observed to affect the mothers' interpretation of symptoms may be compared with Mechanic's concept of 'needs competing with illness response',[4] or Robinson's demonstration, from health diaries, of the influence of family events upon the decision that one of its members is ill.[5] During the six-months' survey it was noted that if the mother had problems at work, or had many other difficulties to contend with, or was moving house, or the child itself had other problems, attention might be directed from the symptoms, which were made to seem trivial in comparison. For instance one mother who worked part-time undoubtedly played down some of her children's problems and sent them to school, because : 'Our boss doesn't like staff staying off work to watch children ... Mine are never off school unless they are dying.' (M12) Her girl of five continued to attend a child-minder during the school holiday, despite bouts of fairly severe tonsillitis: 'I'd no choice. There were two people off on holiday at work.' Again, when a six-months-old baby had 'bad bronchitis' the mother commented:

I maybe should have stayed in with him, but I have to take (four-

and-a-half-year-old daughter) to the nursery and she'd already
been off with mumps ... The girl at the chemist said I shouldn't
be out. I said that I had to go my messages. She said to get a neighbour to do that, but I never see them.(M28)

Another mother, a single parent, had the same problem when her
two year old was recovering from a bad cold in dismal weather;
having been told to keep her in for a week, she found this impossible
since she was on her own, 'So I just wrap her up very well.'(M25)
Another mother who was busy moving house said of her six-year-old
son, who had been 'choking' at night due to a cough: 'I haven't been
to the doctor with him yet. I haven't had time with all this packing.'
(M24)

More attention may, of course, be paid to the symptoms if they
continue to cause the mother a lot of trouble and inconvenience,
such as the great burden of washing created by enuresis and soiling.
Several mothers were distressed by what they termed their children's
'hyperactivity', because it was extremely exhausting for the women
concerned, and some consulted because the children refused to sleep
a full night. M61 eventually became worried about what was usually
seen as a 'normal' problem, e.g. teething, when the whole family lost
sleep and was unable to function normally, saying 'I haven't had a
night's sleep, not one whole night since Christmas.' Other mothers
came to take symptoms seriously when they were 'fed up of the
whining', or 'annoyed by his girning'. Some consultations were
made because the family were due to go on holiday the next day.

It is also possible that children's symptoms were highlighted if
they were believed to be *productive* in some way, in order to bring
about some action which the mother desired. Mothers who wished
their children to have a tonsillectomy perhaps tended to consult more
frequently about sore throats. Others who were anxious to obtain a
new house might also emphasise symptoms. M14 continually
stressed the seriousness of her toddler's 'chest trouble' because she
was desperate to move from a damp and 'undesirable' house, though
the interviewer never heard him cough over the six months. Similarly
M30 had a tendency to emphasise her children's chest conditions and
a lengthy list of other symptoms, as she was also keen to move from
an obviously damp house. One mother who generally paid scant
attention to symptoms sought advice, when she was in a very
advanced state of pregnancy, about her daughter's German measles;
however, she made it very clear that she knew the unborn baby
would not be harmed at this stage, but hoped that the infection
might provide a reason for induction, because she was 'fed up'.

There was also some tendency for the mothers to treat fairly seriously, and take action upon, symptoms which were noted at school or nursery and led to the child being sent home, a letter being sent to the parents, or a phone call from the headmistress. M30 paid particular attention to symptoms which might be noted at school and was always reluctant to send them looking tired or ill:

> You've got to keep yourself right. Cos you can't win, no matter what happens. You've always got somebody on you.

Other examples, among many, were M16 who redefined her child's cold as being more serious when the headmistress sent her home with the diagnosis of measles, and M22 who generally realised that her daughter looked pale and tired, but tended to visit the surgery with her only when a letter appeared from the school nurse to say 'she's not looking well'. Similarly enuresis and soiling noted at school, as opposed simply to 'bed-wetting', tended to be acted upon with greater vigour.

A small number of mothers treated very seriously any symptoms or conditions which 'looked bad' for them, cast aspersions on their hygiene (they believed) and were felt to be stigmatising. For instance, the eczema of M7's two-year-old son had caused arguments and tears at the 'baby clinic' and she became even more anxious to get rid of the problem as holiday time arrived:

> Sometimes it comes up in big red blotches. And I always felt people thought I wasn't looking after him.

M16 immediately telephoned her health visitor when she found 'beasties' in her daughter's hair:

> You see, one evening she was sitting over there scratching her head and she isn't one to scratch. So I looked in her hair and found these things crawling up them. I just panicked. I made her put her head down and used a comb to get them all out. I was going to cut all her hair. But when the health visitor came in she said this was silly and gave me stuff to wash her hair with.(M16)

She (like several others) was very wary about any 'unusual rash':

> Like, I've heard about scabies, but I've never seen it. I've heard you get it from very dirty people—But if there was any rash I didn't recognise I'd call the health visitor right away.(M16)

Reports and Accounts

A description has been given of all the factors which appeared to be important, or which the mothers offered as explanations, in the perception of the children's symptoms over the six months. Obviously, a number of symptoms may not have been reported at all. They might have been noticed by the mother, and then forgotten or not thought worthy of mention. The interviewers occasionally perceived symptoms such as obvious coughs which were never discussed, and the children themselves sometimes called attention to conditions (usually trivial) which their mothers had not mentioned.

The fact that some symptoms may have been noticed but not reported must, of course, be related to the definitions of health and illness described in chapter 4. The condition may have seemed so 'normal' that it need not be reported, and the feeling that illness was a type of failure may have influenced some mothers. Certain conditions may also have been minimised because they were felt to carry an element of stigma: in some cases enuresis was consistently presented as urinary infection or a 'chill'.

It is also extremely difficult to distinguish the 'real' perceptions of the mothers, especially of symptoms not treated seriously, from 'accounts' offered to interviewers as excuses for the actions taken or not taken. The women may have felt that they were being judged in some way, although every effort was made to avoid giving this impression, and consequently may have attempted to normalise symptoms or justify their actions. For instance, motives were frequently imputed to children in order to account for symptoms being interpreted as non-serious:

> It wasn't anything—she probably made herself sick to get off school.(M71)
> She's playing on it. She doesn't want to go to school although she's well enough.(M12)
> But he often makes himself sick if he doesn't get his own way.(M20)
> I think it's [bed-wetting] just laziness. He used to rise during the night, but now he's too lazy in the cold weather.(M20)

It would obviously be unreasonable, however, to present the young mothers as obliged to be perfectly rational about their rules for defining illness, or to suggest that they would always have clear-cut explanations to offer for their help-seeking decisions. Determining whether a child is ill is not always easy, whatever the family's circumstances. Deciding whether or not the illness merits a consultation with a doctor involves another set of factors—such as the accessibility of services or relationships with the medical profession—which may present special difficulties for some families. Attitudes to doctors, and the structure of different services which was available, are topics dealt with in subsequent chapters. This chapter would not be complete, however, without some discussion of the ways in which the mothers' interpretations of symptoms influenced their help-seeking behaviour.

Perception of Symptoms and Consulting Behaviour

Several of the young mothers expressed distress and worry at their own feelings of inadequacy in interpreting symptoms:

> My problem is not *knowing* when I should call [doctor]. If it turns out nothing you just feel you're bothering them.(M61)

Several also ruefully discussed the well-known tendency for small children to recover just before the doctor arrived, or lose their rash or pain at the surgery door. Decisions that 'this is an illness, and serious enough to warrant professional treatment' were not necessarily taken quickly or lightly: for many of the illness episodes reported, there was a long story of indecision and reinterpretation. The grandmother or other lay advisers were consulted, the mother waited until her husband came home, the child seemed to improve so that consultation was delayed, only to become worse again so that the delay was regretted.

Over-quick consultation or delayed consultation might both result in conflict with the doctor. An example of delay might be the mother who waited a day or two when her baby had a high temperature, consulting only when he developed a cough, to be told sharply that 'I should have taken him before'. Over-anxiousness, on the other hand, was very reasonably explained by one of the grandmothers:

> But when the doctor comes in he says, Och, it's a' right—we ken this kinda thing happens. But, I mean, *I* dinna ken this kinda thing happens. Well, I suppose I div ken within mysel' that it dis happen, but I mean—I'm thinking on him, ken? Could they dee somethin' to help him? So naturally you're goin' to send for the doctor, ken?(G30)

The typical reactions to symptoms which have been described obviously had some relevance to both the 'neglect' and 'consultation for trivialities' as professionals might define them. Conditions which were normalised, in a context of low expectations, might represent neglect; ear infections are a prominent example. If the cause of a condition was 'known', and it was thought to be a family weakness or something about which little could be done, again it might be neglected.

On the other hand, it has been noted that the medical history of a particular child might make the mother especially anxious, and she might consult repeatedly about symptoms which had proved to be serious in the past or were suggestive of conditions which had handicapped members of older generations. Some mothers were unusually conscious of the possibility of TB, and many over-emphasised the less serious infectious diseases. Several doctors were reported to have been a little irritable at being called out, as an emergency, to cases of rubella. The account of one mother was:

[Although it was Sunday she asked the doctor to call:] He said, 'Oh, it's just German measles, there's a lot of it about', and I said 'Well, I'm worried and I don't see how you can diagnose it over the phone.' He said 'Who am I talking to?' and I said 'It's Mrs [64] and can I ask your name as well?' Eventually he said he'd call. Then ten minutes later rang back and said he couldn't come, he'd been called out to an emergency, it was all dramatical like, saving someone's life with a burst ulcer. But eventually he said he'd see me if I came to the surgery [which was opened specially. The diagnosis was in fact German measles.]

In situations of conflict, when the mothers thought they were being accused of fussing or being over-demanding, they frequently appealed to their own special knowledge of the child. If they were wrong about the importance of the symptoms, they found it difficult to explain to doctors why they acted as they did.

Obviously, there were other more practical factors which influenced the decision to consult or not about a given symptom. Some mothers consulted frequently, simply because the surgery was so convenient, or the clinic did not necessitate an appointment. Others asked for home visits because of a long distance to the surgery, the problem of taking a sick child out in cold weather or on buses, or difficulties about looking after other children. The difference between the 'more' and the 'less' disadvantaged noted on p. 48 is largely accounted for in this way. A few of the 'more' disadvantaged mothers who were 'low consulters' may—because of their more difficult life circumstances—have been slightly less ready to notice symptoms in their children, or had lower standards of normal health. This possibility applies to only a small number, however. For the most part, the 'less' disadvantaged were likely to consult more only because there were fewer obstacles in their way.

References

[1] Zborowski, M. (1952), 'Cultural components in response to pain', *J. Soc. Issues*, **8**, 16.
Zola, I. K. (1966), 'Culture and symptoms: an analysis of patients' presenting complaints', *Amer. Soc. Rev.*, **31**, 615.

[2] Di Cocco, L. and Apple, D. (1960), 'Health needs and symptoms of older adults' in Apple, D. (ed.), *Sociological Studies of Health and Sickness*, New York: McGraw-Hill.

Gordon, G. (1966), *Role Theory and Illness*, New Haven: College and University Press.

[3] Koos, E. L. (1954), *The Health of Regionsville*, New York: Columbia University Press.

Zola, I. K. (1964), 'Illness behaviour of the working class' in Shostak, A. and Gomberg, W. (eds.), *Blue Collar World*, Englewood Cliff, N.J.: Prentice-Hall.

Alpert, J. J., Kosa, J. and Haggerty, R. J. (1967), 'A month of illness and health care among low income families', *Public Health Reports*, **82**, 8, 705.

Rainwater, L. (1968), 'The lower class: health, illness and medical institutions' in Deutscher, I. and Thompson, E. J. (eds.), *Among the People: Encounters with the Poor*, New York: Basic Books.

Cartwright, A. and O'Brien, M. (1976), 'Social class variations in health care and the nature of general practice consultations' in Stacey, M. (ed.), *The Sociology of the NHS*, London: Croom Helm.

Campbell, J. D. (1978), 'The child in the sick role: contributions of age, sex, parental status and parental values', *J. Health Soc. Behav.*, **19**, 35.

[4] Mechanic, D. (1968), *Medical Sociology*. New York: Free Press.

[5] Robinson, D. (1971), *The Process of Becoming Ill*. London: Routledge and Kegan Paul.

7 Chronic and Handicapping Conditions among the Children

Although there was no evidence that the majority of the children of our families suffered from more incidents of acute illness than the average, it did seem that an unduly high proportion did suffer from chronic problems of various sorts. It also seemed that it was in connection with these chronic conditions that service-use was most likely to be full of conflict. Chronic problems were therefore submitted to a detailed analysis, based on the evidence of written records and of health visitors, as well as the systematic recording of events over six months.

Prevalence of Chronic Conditions among the Children
Of our 139 children, we judged that 65 suffered *currently* from chronic conditions or handicaps, with a slightly greater proportion of boys than of girls. Only those conditions which troubled the children throughout the six-months' survey, or are permanent handicaps, are included in Table 7.1. This is not a record of all the chronic conditions *ever* suffered, and now cured, which would of course be much longer. We believe that we have, from records and the mothers' accounts, a fairly complete list of all the serious illnesses in the children's history, but we cannot be sure of this, and for events in the past there are inevitably problems about precise diagnoses or definitions of seriousness.

The children may also seem to the mothers to have current problems which have not been diagnosed, and these too have been omitted since we could not make judgements about them. For conditions such as speech or behaviour disorder, or enuresis, which may apply in minor degrees to many children, we have avoided problems of definition by including only those which had been brought to professional attention and clinically identified as being serious enough to require investigation or treatment.

Our small numbers, and the fact that we are considering children of all ages up to 12, makes it difficult to compare this record of chronic disease with larger epidemiological studies. It would appear,

Table 7.1   Diagnosed chronic conditions among the children

	M	F	Both
Children with one or more chronic condition	35 (51%)	30 (43%)	65 (47%)
Children without chronic conditions	34 (49%)	40 (57%)	74 (53%)
(N = 100%)	(69)	(70)	(139)

Conditions suffered, numbers of children

	M	F
Chronic otitis media	8	5
Deafness, partial or total	2	—
Squint	5	6
Other eye disorder	3	2
Chronic bronchitis	5	3
TB (effects of)	1	1
Heart murmur	2	1
Crippling conditions	2	1
Asthma	2	—
Anaemia	—	2
Eczema	3	2
Epilepsy	—	1
Convulsions (not more specifically diagnosed)	2	2
Chronic headache	1	2
Chronic urinary infection	—	6
Enuresis/incontinence (serious enough to have been treated)	8	5
Speech defect (clinically diagnosed and treated)	5	—
Behaviour problem (referred to child psychologist)	2	2
Mental handicap	1	—

however, that the rate in our families of *present* otitis media—9.36 per cent—was similar to that found in the National Child Development Survey (NCDS) for *past and present* otitis media in social class V children at seven years, 9.57 per cent.[1] The rate of ever having had otitis media by seven was certainly very much higher in our children: bearing in mind that we may not have a full record, it appeared to be at least 18 per cent. The condition, at the present time, was sufficiently severe in our children for nine of the 13 cases to have had the surgical insertion of grommets for drainage. Similarly, a prevalence of squint at seven years for children of social class V of 3.48 per cent was reported in the NCDS. The prevalence of squint among our children was 7.9 per cent.

For some conditions, the rates of recorded defects at school entry in overall Scottish statistics may be compared, although these deal with one age-cohort of children whereas our sample is of varied ages. In 1978, the rates of enuresis found in school entrants was 5.6 per cent (boys) and 4.9 per cent (girls). 'Inflammatory condition of the ear' was found in about 1 per cent of children and 'strabismus' in about 3 per cent.[2] The tentative comparisons which can be made therefore all suggest that there was an unduly high prevalence of chronic conditions among this sample of children.

Adverse birth conditions

An accurate record of conditions associated with the birth of the children was available from maternity hospital records, as well as from the mothers' accounts. Since these may be relevant to the children's subsequent health, they are listed in Table 7.2.

The problem of defining those conditions which are significant is avoided by including only those which resulted in the infant being cared for in the Special Nursery of the maternity hospital. We have no evidence of adverse birth conditions in any infant *not* so treated. The rate of 26 per cent may be compared with the rate of admission to the Special Nursery of all children born in the City during the

Table 7.2 Significant adverse birth conditions

	M		F		Both	
Children with adverse birth condition	18	(26%)	18	(26%)	36	(26%)
Children without adverse birth condition	51	(74%)	52	(74%)	103	(74%)
(N = 100%)	(69)		(70)		(139)	

Conditions, numbers of children

	M	F
LBW or light-for-dates	6	7
Premature	4	2
Forceps delivery	2	3
Jaundice	5	—
Asphyxia	3	1

And three or fewer cases each of: antepartum haemorrhage, foetal distress, hypothermia, cyanotic attack, breech delivery, clicking hip, skin sepsis, vomiting, failure to feed, mother diabetic, mother TB, and at risk of hereditary disease.

(One child may be listed for more than one condition)

1970s—varying, of course, over time but roughly 12–15 per cent.

The children included rather high proportions who were illegitimate (13.7 per cent), prenuptially conceived (24.5 per cent) and/or born to very young mothers (14.2 per cent to mothers aged 18 or younger). Since the children are now of all ages up to 12, it is not easy to provide comparable figures for the population from which the sample is drawn. However, in the City in the year 1970, 8 per cent of births in all social classes were illegitimate, and 8 per cent were to mothers aged 18 and younger.

The relationship between these factors, adverse birth conditions, and the health status of the children at the present time is shown in Table 7.3.

Table 7.3 Relationship of birth status, age of mother at delivery, and adverse birth conditions, with chronic ill health now

	Chronic conditions now		No chronic condition now		N (= 100%)
Birth status:					
Illegitimate	11	(59%)	8	(41%)	19
Prenuptial conception	17	(50%)	17	(50%)	34
Conceived within marriage	37	(43%)	49	(57%)	86
Age of mother at delivery:					
18 and under	13	(48%)	14	(52%)	27
19 and over	52	(46%)	60	(54%)	112
Adverse birth condition:					
Condition listed in Table 7.2	21	(58%)	15	(42%)	36
No adverse birth condition	43	(42%)	60	(58%)	103

Of course all these may be associated. Illegitimate and prenuptial conceptions are likely to be to younger mothers: they included all but two of the births at 18 and under, but only 25 per cent of the births at 19 and over. Adverse birth conditions are also more likely among young mothers (see Table 7.4).

Table 7.4 Relationship of age of mother at delivery with adverse birth conditions

	Adverse birth conditions		No adverse birth conditions		N (= 100%)
Age of mother at delivery:					
18 and under	10	(37%)	17	(63%)	27
19 and over	26	(23%)	86	(77%)	112

Infant morbidity

Another factor which may be associated both with adverse birth conditions, and with chronic ill health later in childhood, is morbidity in infancy. Children who suffer some particular conditions in their early years have been shown to be more likely to experience ill health throughout childhood.[3] We have therefore extracted from the children's health records (which are fuller and more likely to be reliable in the first few years than in the later years of childhood) the conditions which we believe may be significant, in the history of all the children now of two years and over (see Table 7.5).

Table 7.5 Significant morbidity under two years of age

	M	F	Both
Suffered infant morbidity	24 (44%)	22 (34%)	46 (39%)
No infant morbidity	31 (56%)	42 (66%)	73 (61%)
(N = 100%) (children now of 2 years and over)	(55)	(64)	(119)

Conditions suffered, numbers of children

	M	F
Measles	6	4
Otitis media	2	3
Pneumonia	2	2
Bronchitis	7	4
Repeated diarrhoea and vomiting; gastroenteritis; dysentery	7	9
'Failure to thrive'; clinical concern about care	3	9

Also, one or two cases each of: scarlet fever, whooping cough, TB, mumps, anaemia, meningitis, jaundice, hiatus hernia, coeliac disease (diagnosis queried), pyelonephritis, pyloric stenosis, nephrectomy, and non-accidental injury.

(One child may have suffered more than one condition)

Table 7.6 shows that these children were indeed more likely to have chronic conditions now than were children who had not suffered from any of the listed conditions during their first two years.

Some of this association may be direct and causal, but in most cases there seemed to be no direct connection between the specific infant illness and the present chronic condition. Of the ten children who had infant measles, four had no chronic conditions now, and two had obviously unconnected conditions. Of the 11 children who had infant bronchitis, only one had a chronic chest condition now,

Table 7.6   Relationship of infant morbidity and chronic conditions now (children aged 2 and over)

	Chronic condition now	No chronic condition now	N (= 100%)
Infant morbidity:			
Suffered condition			
listed in Table 7.5	28 (61%)	18 (39%)	46
Did not	32 (44%)	41 (56%)	73

six had other chronic conditions and four had no chronic conditions. In this sample, it appeared that it is rather deficiency in general health represented by serious illness in infancy which is either the cause of, or is an indicator of the likelihood of, continued childhood ill health.

Relationship with social disadvantage

These associations are complicated, of course, by the fact that adverse birth conditions may make infant morbidity more likely, and that both of these—and continuing ill health—may be associated with particularly adverse social conditions. It appears from Table 7.7

Table 7.7   Relationship of adverse birth conditions and infant morbidity with index of 'disadvantage' of the family

Child in family which is:	Adverse birth conditions Yes	No	Infant morbidity Yes	No	N (= 100%)
'More disadvantaged'	24 (31%)	53 (69%)	30 (39%)	47 (61%)	77
'Less disadvantaged'	12 (19%)	50 (81%)	16 (26%)	46 (74%)	62

that adverse birth conditions, and morbidity under two years of age, are more likely to characterise families in our 'more disadvantaged' group than in the 'less disadvantaged' (see Appendix B). It must be noted that this index is based on the families' circumstances *now*, rather than at the previous time when these events occurred. Obviously there is some likelihood of the index selecting families whose childbearing did start off in disadvantaged circumstances, though it may exclude some who had become more prosperous and stable despite a bad start.

From Table 7.8, however, it seems that the prevalence of chronic conditions in the children now is not very strongly associated with disadvantaged circumstances now, despite the association of 'disadvantage' at the present time and illegitimate births, youthful conceptions and adverse birth conditions. This is, of course, a comparison between the more and less disadvantaged *within* our sample.

Considering this social class IV/V group *as a whole*, in comparison with the rest of the population, we have already indicated that the prevalence of the sort of chronic conditions found is probably high compared to that in more fortunate social classes.

Table 7.8 Relationship of index of 'disadvantage' of the family with chronic conditions now

	Chronic conditions now	No chronic conditions now	N (= 100%)
Child in family which is:			
'More disadvantaged'	34 (44%)	43 (56%)	77
'Less disadvantaged'	31 (50%)	31 (50%)	62

'At Risk' Registers

The child health service caring for these children had, like most others, a system of 'At Risk' registration in operation. The utility of such registers, and the principles by which children should be chosen to be placed on them, have been matters of some dispute.[4] Whether or not a child is labelled 'At Risk', with the implication of special monitoring of development, is obviously relevant in the context of congenital or chronic conditions and handicaps.

A high proportion of our children, 24 per cent, were designated 'At Risk' at some time. The criteria which were applied locally for placement on the register changed during the period represented by the birth dates of the children, but about half of the registrations were on medical grounds only (birth conditions or events in early infancy) and about half on social grounds (illegitimacy, disturbed family history) either alone or together with medical criteria. We cannot, of course, say what the precise reasons for the child's being selected were in every case, since such a decision has to be taken by individuals and we cannot know what factors were being taken into account at the time. More first-born children (36 per cent) than subsequently born (17 per cent of second and 8 per cent of third) were designated 'At Risk' (since they were more likely to be illegitimate, have very young mothers, and/or to suffer adverse birth conditions).

Looking simply at the known circumstances of the children's births or infancy it is sometimes difficult to understand why certain children were *not*, according to the available records, placed on the register. Most illegitimate children who had very adverse medical conditions at birth were, but a proportion remained who were not. An example might be a child (now three) who had been cared for in the Special Nursery because light-for-dates, who had suffered from hypothermia, vomiting and failure to feed, and whose parents were living at the time in one room.

The efficiency of the register in selecting children may be considered by noting the relationship of the 'At Risk' group to the larger group who, at the present time, have handicaps or chronic conditions. Table 7.9 suggests that the 'At Risk' procedure was reasonably efficient in the sense that it selected only a relatively small group (27 per cent) who had in fact had no continuing health problems. On the other hand, it must be noted that only 37 per cent of the 65 children who did have problems were selected as 'At Risk'.

Table 7.9 Relationship of designation as 'At Risk' with existence of chronic conditions now

	Chronic condition now	No chronic condition now	N (= 100%)
'At Risk'	24 (73%)	9 (27%)	33
Not 'At Risk'	41 (39%)	65 (61%)	106

It has already been shown that children with adverse birth conditions, and those who were illegitimate and/or had very young mothers, and those who suffered certain types of morbidity in their first two years, are more likely to be amongst those who had chronic conditions at the time of the survey. Those who were, and were not, selected as 'At Risk' may be compared. Except for the illegitimacy/young mother category, we cannot of course do the same for the 'social' criteria: we have no objective way of measuring 'poor social circumstances' at the time of a particular child's birth years ago, and the fact that there is no mention in the records of particularly adverse circumstances does not necessarily mean that there were none.

Table 7.10 seems to suggest that 'adverse birth conditions', when identified as an 'At Risk' characteristic, were efficient in selecting the children who continued to have troubled health, although there remained 19 per cent of the children who did have adverse birth conditions who were not selected and who—in hindsight—might profitably have been. The conclusion with regard to illegitimacy and/or young mothers (not, of course, independent of the other adverse conditions) is similar. It appears, however, that the conditions listed in Table 7.5 as significant infant morbidity, less frequently selected as grounds for designation as 'At Risk', might profitably be given more consideration—whether alone or together with other factors—as meriting the continued special monitoring of the children.

Table 7.10 Relationship of adverse circumstances, designation as 'At Risk' and chronic conditions now

	Chronic conditions now		No chronic condition now		N
	Designated 'At Risk'	Not designated 'At Risk'	Designated 'At Risk'	Not designated 'At Risk'	(=100%)
Adverse birth condition (Table 7.2)	14 (39%)	7 (19%)	6 (17%)	9 (25%)	36
Significant infant morbidity (Table 7.5)	12 (26%)	16 (35%)	3 (13%)	15 (33%)	46
Illegitimate and/or mother 18 years and under	15 (41%)	5 (13%)	4 (11%)	13 (35%)	37
Children with both					
(a) Illegitimate and/or mother 18 years and under *and*					
(b) adverse birth conditions and/or infant morbidity	12 (60%)	3	2	3	20

Individual children may of course appear in more than one of these categories. We are considering here the children's actual circumstances, not those which were the apparent grounds for placing on the 'At Risk' register. In the case of infant morbidity in particular, children may have come into this category after having been placed on the register.

There are, of course, several ways of interpreting these data. It may be argued that the 'At Risk' register, with all the idiosyncracies of decision making that are inevitable, and despite changes during the period of ten years or so which is relevant, has been reasonably efficient in selecting out those children who were likely to have health problems. Those children on the register who are healthy now may have had problems in the past, now cured. On the other hand, the objective of such a register is to prevent handicap as far as possible, or at least to monitor and manage in the most effective way any health deficit which is inevitable. From this point of view the fact that a high proportion of these children still have problems may (depending on the nature of these conditions) be disturbing. The identification and management of chronic conditions is obviously relevant.

The Management of Chronic Problems

The management of the children's acute episodes of illness was, it has been suggested, variable in what might be considered a very 'normal' way—sometimes problematic to the mothers, and sometimes straightforward; likely to be stressful in certain circumstances or for some families, but generally dealt with without a great deal of trouble. Relationships with health-service personnel might similarly exhibit conflict for some people or in some situations, but for the most part the mothers obtained the service they felt they needed, in one way or another. Our impression of the management of chronic conditions, however, was that this must give more cause for concern. Of the families with handicaps or long-term conditions generally, there were few who were untroubled about their relationships with health services.

In discussing the reasons for this, we must inevitably be dealing to some extent with anecdotal material. We do not imply that everything we were told must be objectively true. Mothers might forget, exaggerate, or confuse the timing of what had happened. In relating events over, perhaps, many years it would be surprising if the mothers had not—without any intentional misrepresentation—rewritten their stories, and re-interpreted the past in the light of what they knew now. Various methods of checking were open to us, such as the examination of records and the comparison of the independent account of grandmothers and mothers. As far as the events occurring during the survey period are concerned, we believe we have accurate accounts. In general, however, we present these data only as a description of how the mothers *perceived* events, and what the consequences were.

The recognition and diagnosis of chronic conditions

The first point of conflict for our mothers concerned the belief of many of them that they had noticed a possible handicap in a child, or the symptoms of a chronic condition, which they insist they brought to the notice of doctors—perhaps many times—before they could 'get it taken seriously', and long before diagnostic investigations were undertaken. For instance, one mother's account of the identification of mental handicap in her son was that the grandmother first noticed that something was wrong because 'he would never look you in the eye', and though their fears were mentioned to the doctor and health visitor they were told there was nothing wrong: 'They said that all children do things in their own time. But they were never with him long enough. He looked normal to them.' The child's records confirm that the first specialist assessment was made when he was two, although there are previous comments noting that the mother was concerned about his development. This mother was insistent that no one would tell her *why* the boy was handicapped, perhaps because it had only been investigated at two: 'Maybe they would if it had happened at birth. I suppose it *did* happen at birth but it wasn't noticed.' This child was premature and a forceps delivery, the mother had been ill throughout pregnancy, and the family circumstances then (though not now) were very disturbed: the boy had been on the 'At Risk' register from birth.

A similar story was told by the mother of a six-year-old boy whose crippling condition was the cause of much concern and disability during our survey period, who reported having been told by doctors 'to ignore it, he would grow out of it'. The notes on this child, who had a clicking hip at birth and was also on the 'At Risk' register, certainly contained no mention of any query about his condition until during his third year.

A final example is another boy, now five, with many operations upon his eye, who was waiting for further surgery during the survey period. The mother insisted that a squint was first noticed at five months, but the health visitor's notes first mentioned it at $1\frac{1}{2}$ years. Again, the mother believed that this and other troubles that the boy suffered might be due to a very difficult birth, but felt that she had to fight to get the seriousness of his handicap recognised.

It does seem possible that mothers (and grandmothers) may, out of their particular knowledge of their children, recognise abnormalities before clear clinical diagnoses can be given. Several indicated to us that they thought that instincts of this sort had been brushed aside. Of course, we are more likely to have heard of the cases where these feelings proved well-grounded: there may have been many worries which were needless, of which we never heard. Also, it is possible that the children's handicaps could not have been diagnosed earlier, and it is, of course, part of medical management not to alarm parents until certainty has been reached, or until the time has arrived when some treatment may be possible. We cannot have the accounts of the doctors concerned, who might include many individuals both inside and outside hospitals over many years. It might well be that the cases were being managed in full recognition of all the possibilities, and the mothers were mistaken in thinking that they were not. Nor have we any clear evidence that the children were harmed by what the mothers saw as delay and inattention. What is certain, however, is that the mothers' relationships with health services became full of conflict.

Conflict over the management of chronic conditions

The consequences of conflict over identification, and over the subsequent management of chronic conditions, could be very unfortunate. If it seemed to the mothers that 'nothing is being done', this might well be transformed into 'no one will take this seriously'. The mother might feel that she was not being believed, that she was being labelled as a 'fusser', or that 'nobody cares'. The result might be anger, displayed in a desperate thrashing about for attention, or it might be apathy and the avoidance of contact with health services.

One mother, for instance, said that she had tried for three years to persuade her doctor that her daughter was deaf, but he had said that there was nothing wrong, 'he said she just didn't want to hear'. The results of eventual treatment had not been successful, and now the mother believed that a second child 'is going the same way' but she had not mentioned it to her doctor, because she would be 'worried about her going into hospital in case the same thing happened'.

Another mother had experienced serious difficulties with a child's eczema from the time when he was three months old until after he was three (confirmed by the health visitor's records). She felt that this had never been taken seriously, and after one occasion when, following an argument at the child health clinic, she had (according to the health visitor's notes) 'left weeping', she refused to return to the clinic.

Similarly, in the case of a seven-year-old girl with enuresis, the mother said at the beginning of the survey period that although the child was attending a hospital clinic, she did not find it very helpful: 'It's a waste of time, they just speak, they don't *do* anything' and two months later she said, after another visit: 'If they won't do anything, I'm not going back. I've been going back now for six years.' She did not keep her next appointment.

Of course the mothers' perception that 'nothing is being done' may have resulted from the simple fact that there was nothing, at a particular stage, which *could* be done. The health visitor commented about the case of enuresis:

> Well, they can't really do very much. They can only see if there's no urine infection and give her some support. If it's a familial thing she'll just grow out of it.

Enuresis and squints were, in fact, two conditions about which there was commonly the greatest conflict. The problem about squints was not only that the time had to be appropriate for treatment, but also that the mothers believed that there was a long waiting list.

These two conditions were ones which were seen, by several health visitors at least, as almost normal among the children living in the poorest areas. The health visitor quoted above had described enuresis as 'familial' and believed that the problem was 'passed down' within families. There was also some indication of the mothers being given very stereotyped explanations for enuresis, which they—quite sensibly, in many cases—found inadequate; it seemed that their very real and individual problem was not being given individual consideration. The enuresis of one five-year-old boy, for instance, must—the doctors suggested—be a disturbance due to jealousy of his younger sister. His mother thought that several other factors might be relevant: that the child had sustained a birth injury, had had many operations on his eyes, had poor balance and was accident-prone, was having many problems with schoolwork, and had begun to exhibit enuresis at the time when he knew he was going back into hospital for further surgery.

Communication failures

In these cases where the management of chronic conditions was full of conflict, it seemed that at the least communication had been faulty. It was in fact lack of information, rather than any allegations about actual treatment, that was the most common complaint. The

mothers were almost unanimous in their praise of everyone concerned when their children were inpatients in the children's hospital,
but they felt very differently about outpatient clinics. Their
expectations of clinics were that they were the place where decisions
were taken about treatment, where diagnoses and prognoses were
pronounced upon, and where all their worries could be discussed.
The clinic appointments were important events to most mothers, and
might involve a great deal of practical trouble in taking time off
work and arranging for the care of other children. In the event, of
course, their expectations were rarely met, and they complained of
long waits, hurried consultations, and—especially—lack of information.

One description was:

> It's horrible, you go into a room and there's two men speaking
> over your head, really they're rude for that. [She was given a pre-
> scription but] he wisnae going to tell me what it was for. I was just
> supposed to throw it down his throat.

And another mother commented:

> The inpatients are very good ... they're very good to the kids,
> plenty of time, plenty of patience ... But at the outpatients, it was
> a disappointing service, ken. You've to sit aboot for hours. An'
> then they'll tell you you're not supposed to be there that day. And
> if you do go on the right day, you still sit aboot for hours. And
> they're calling this doctor and they're calling that doctor, and
> they're never anywhere to be found.

And on another occasion, concerning another child, at a different
department of the hospital:

> If you go in, the doctor'll say, Oh yes, X-ray. That's all he does,
> until the X-ray comes back. And then he looks at the X-rays, and
> he'll say, Keep the cast on another week. And that's it. You've sat
> about there, just to be told to keep the cast on another week. [And
> of another doctor] He was very abrupt. It costs nothing to be nice,
> or even polite, ken. It's a case of 'go for the X-ray' and 'Oh, aye,
> nothing there, take him away for six months, he'll grow out of
> it' ... one hand doesna ken fit [know what] the other hand's
> doing ... it sickens you.

There were some indications that, in what they perceived as rushed
and stressful encounters, the mothers could easily misunderstand or
forget anything that they *had* been told. One had been consulting
about a boy's chronic gastrointestinal complaint. She was very
unsure of the diagnosis she had been given after one particular consultation, and in reply to the question 'Did you understand? What
do you think the doctor meant?', she replied:

I'm not sure now. I thought it seemed sense at the time! [Did he give you detailed instructions?] You know, I don't mind [remember] exactly what he said. But I know what I have to do, give him things that don't make him run—I'm careful about vegetables and that. [On a later occasion, after she had decided that this was quite the wrong thing to have done:] Sheer ignorance, it was. I see it now—I thought I was doing the right thing and I wisnae.

On the occasions when mothers did meet what they saw as consideration and careful explanation, they were extremely grateful to the individual doctors concerned. One mother expressed this well, and also demonstrated that she understood clearly the organisational reasons why such a consultation was rare:

... it wis him that sat doon and explained everything to me aboot this dyslexia or fitever it is, he's good like that, because he disnae need to tak' time to tell me a' that, that's nae his job, he's only there for eyes, ken. [She went on to say that this creates long waits, however, because] he forgets, ken, that there's only five minutes atween appointments, once he starts telling you something he gets so inveigled in it he's got to gie ye the hale story—he mak's the appointments a' run late. But he's good like that.

This same mother had previously been eloquent about what seemed to her a reluctance to give her any explanations of what was happening, from the time of the child's birth onwards:

Just, oh, he's fine, that was all they telt you—I asked whit it wis an' naebody says—they dinna believe in giein' ye that much information.

She was only one among many who expressed very particular distress over lack of information while the newborn child was being cared for in the Special Nursery. It appeared to them that their own care, and the care of the child, were being separated and they did not know who to approach for information. Often they thought that nurses might be more approachable, but for obvious reasons they found that their inquiries were greeted with evasions and sometimes conflicting information.

The mothers' most desperately expressed needs as the child grew up were for explanations, or at least discussions, of *why* the child was like this. Sometimes they recognised that a clear diagnosis might not be possible—though often they believed that a diagnosis must have been made, and they were being kept in ignorance. One mother worried at length about the cause of her four-year-old child's frequent convulsions and hyperactivity. Could it have been due to the child's prematurity? The fact that the mother was 'very ill and sick the whole pregnancy'? The rash 'which they thought might be measles' which she had had during pregnancy? The child's whooping-cough injection? She said:

> The doctors talk among themselves. They would talk past you if you didn't speak to them . . . They don't give anything away. I think they're scared to.

During the survey period this mother surreptitiously read the child's file while she was at her general practitioner's surgery, and noted a diagnosis of epilepsy:

> And the hospital say they don't know why he takes fits! I would have thought we would have been told. I wouldn't have known if I hadn't seen it written down. If it's that, he could take them at any time. The last fit wasn't connected with an illness. If he's epileptic he might not grow out of it.

In these comments she was explaining clearly why it was that she felt she needed to know the diagnosis. It was relevant for the handling of the child, because she had thought before that she needed to watch him carefully only when he had minor infections. Also, she had been told comfortingly that he 'would grow out of it', but now she felt that her whole view of her family's future might have to change.

Again, both mother and grandparents were very concerned about a precise diagnosis and prognosis for a mentally handicapped boy. Mental handicap meant, to the mother, lack of intelligence. Yet both she and the grandparents felt this was not entirely an appropriate label, for in some ways the boy did not seem to them to be stupid:

> A lot of the time he seems intelligent. He talks about the sun and the moon—things other kids wouldn't think about. And he'll ask question after question. Like in the butchers, he said 'Who put the blood in the liver?' How can you answer that? I just say 'God' now. [She said that she did not think that the doctors really knew what was wrong with him, but] I think they should tell you what their thoughts are. In case they are wrong and they don't want to be wrong. Maybe that's why they don't tell you.

Interrelation of services

One of the most common complaints relevant to this feeling about a lack of clear information was of seeing 'a different doctor every time' at outpatient clinics. Many other individuals might be involved also—general practitioners and child health clinic doctors, health visitors and school health services, and specialist therapists of various sorts. If it seemed to the mothers that they were receiving conflicting information, or if they did not understand the organisational processes or the professional etiquette which dictated modes of referral, then it seemed to them that they were caught in a labyrinth. They were not sure, amongst all the people involved, which path led where, or where final responsibility lay. Also, they frequently felt that communication between different parts of the system was poor, and that their attempts to act as go-between or to reconcile seemingly different views only put them into difficult positions. For instance, one mother was concerned because her son's head teacher was keeping him back a year because his sight was, she said, affecting his school work:

> At the hospital they say it's rubbish, that he can see ... I told [the head teacher] that she wasn't an eye specialist and the specialist says his eye-sight is OK. [Nevertheless the child was kept back, and when the mother told the specialist about it] ... he went mad, and said his sight is better than average.

The mother was told to ask to see an educational psychologist—but not to go through the school, but through her general practitioner. There were occasional clashes between the school and other health services, or between the school and the parents, in some other cases, such as when children appeared to have been referred to speech therapists without the parents being informed. One mother found herself at a loss when the teachers of the special school which her son attended rejected the only label for his handicap—autism—which the doctors had offered. We also had accounts of what the mothers felt to be conflicts between the hospital and the general practitioner, sometimes because the family doctor said that he had not been given some particular piece of information from the hospital.

The results of what appeared to be a fragmented service were unfortunate in perhaps two ways. First, to the mothers—who of course saw their children as individuals with problems which were necessarily interrelated—it might seem that each aspect of the child's health and development was being treated separately, with the essential connections ignored. The mother quoted on p. 80 knew that the hearing problems, and the speech problems, and the 'nervousness' of one of her sons were connected ('He doesn't like meeting people. He knows he can't speak properly'), as another knew that her son's eye-operations, enuresis, and learning problems could not be separated. They felt, however, that learning and behaviour difficulties in particular were taken out of their proper context, and separated from the medical condition which might be the cause.

Secondly, there were cases where it seemed that a multiplicity of services, involving very many people, might have been one reason why some handicaps, once identified, were apparently never followed up or adequately treated. Obviously, this would only occur in the few cases where the mother herself did not seem to appreciate what was wrong and so initiated no action herself. In one such case a complicating factor had been that the mother had moved, so that health visitor contact was lost, just as the child was starting school. This seven-year-old boy had a noticeable squint, possible hearing loss, and very poor speech. Lack of treatment for these conditions was certainly not due to an absence of identifying services. A first health visitor had noted the mother's worries because the child had no speech at 15 months. A second had noted a squint, and still no speech, at 2 years. During the child's first year the mother attended a clinic (though infrequently: 7 visits were noted) where the squint was recorded. At another clinic, to which there were two visits during the child's second year, a hearing loss was noticed. At $2\frac{1}{2}$ the child had attended a hearing clinic, where a hearing loss was diagnosed, and at 3 the squint and poor speech were noted at a developmental assessment. The parents were divorced during the child's third year, and since the mother returned to work the boy attended a day nursery, where it was recorded that he had no speech and appeared to be emotionally disturbed. There was no record, nor any account from the mother, of the squint or hearing loss being investigated further. When the child started school he had received treatment from a visiting speech therapist, but this stopped after one year. During the survey period the question of speech therapy was raised again, but since this now meant the mother taking him to the clinic, and her work made it difficult, he attended only a very few times. There is no doubt that this mother, in very difficult social circumstances, had not been particularly active or good at keeping appointments. Nevertheless the child (born prematurely and when the mother was very young) had been on the 'At Risk' register, and had been known to a large number of services: it did seem that perhaps clearer lines of responsibility might have ensured more vigorous follow-up.

Two or three mothers mentioned that, where a child had chronic problems, they found the break with the health visiting service at five years old distressing. We noted that some families had had as many as five different health visitors over five years: in such cases a close relationship might be difficult to establish. There were other mothers, however, who relied very much on a well-known health visitor, and were very disappointed when she gave up visiting when the children started school. It must be added that in fact several health visitors *did* continue to visit children with chronic problems, or were reported to have said to the mother that they would be pleased to speak to her on the telephone at any time.

Conclusion—the Mothers' Needs

This section has focused, for obvious reasons, upon problems and conflicts. Of course, it must not be implied that chronic conditions were *never* managed without stress. The factors which seemed to be most favourable included: the feeling of the mother that she understood the condition, and its cause; her belief that something was being done; having been given, by people she trusted, some grounds for hope; and the mother's confidence that she knew what to do in emergencies and how the condition should best be handled. Anxiety could be relieved by action: the mother whose worries over her child's convulsions were illustrated on p. 81 who had complained that the only person who had ever given her instructions about what to do when the child had an attack was an ambulance attendant, may be contrasted with another, who knew precisely how to handle a child's fits and whose relationship with doctors about them was relatively smooth.

Much of the literature on childhood handicap is concerned with discussions of the concept of stigma, and the possible guilt felt by parents who have a damaged child. We must report that we found very little evidence of any feeling of stigma. Such evidence might have been provided by the mothers, or grandmothers, not mentioning to us conditions which were noted in the records, or by 'disclosures' of more stigmatised conditions being made only in our later interviews, when the mothers might be expected to feel more relaxed and friendly. In fact, neither happened. The mothers appeared to give us true accounts of their children's history, as they perceived it, from the first interview: or if not they achieved the remarkable feat of remembering what they had said six months afterwards. The only impression of a feeling of stigma that we received was in connection with attendance at Special Schools in perhaps two cases, but it was the school which was seen as conferring stigma upon the child, rather than the handicap *per se*.

Nor is guilt an accurate description of the parent's feelings. One health visitor, discussing a mother's conflicts with her doctor over a chronic condition, described her as 'demoralised', and added: 'They feel it is their fault. There's no real fault on either side. They want a perfect baby.' Of course there is a sense in which this must be true, and we would not wish to dismiss the views derived from health visitors' long experience of dealing with families. There have been many studies of mothers' reactions to the birth of a handicapped child, which have demonstrated that feelings of guilt may well be one component of a complex response. None of our families, however, was in the position of having *recently* had a handicapped baby. Our impression of their later reactions is that though parents may 'want a perfect baby', and indeed are very ready to make connections between birth circumstances for which they may take responsibility and subsequent imperfections (as quotations already given may demonstrate), as the baby becomes a child the concept of 'fault' becomes less relevant. The child, to them, is a complex individual, with his own weaknesses and strengths. One mother spoke much more of her worries about current problems with her other children than about her quite severly handicapped eldest son, whose problems were dealt with and stabilised: though handicapped, he was (she insisted) more competent and less troublesome than some of his siblings. From the words which parents used in speaking of their handicapped children, lists of characteristics identifying that child could be derived: they invariably included more positive than negative attributions.

Rather than guilt, it was *responsibility* which they felt so heavily. For an acute emergency, once the decision to place the matter in professional hands was taken, responsibility could be devolved. Where the child had handicaps or chronic conditions continuing for years, however, and given the number of professionals who might be involved, responsibility for making the best choices, ensuring that no avenue of help was overlooked, fighting for the child at every step, remained—the parents felt—with them. Yet at any given point they might be criticised for trying to insert their own special knowledge of the child into the situation or seeming to question decisions made by successive professionals. One was very unsure about the management of her son's sight problem; she acknowledged that her lay observation might be wrong, but it seemed to her that perhaps treatment had been based on false premises. The crucial event had, she thought, been a sight test. On that occasion her interpretation of what had been going on, based on her knowledge of the child and her understanding of why he gave the answers he did, was different to that of the professionals. She said:

> You don't know if you're making the right decision. But if you go against the doctor you're at fault.

Of course, she may well have been quite mistaken. Her words demonstrate clearly, however, the general feeling amongst most of the mothers that ultimately the decisions were theirs: they had an entrepreneurial function and they had to live with the long-term responsibility. It was to exercise this responsibility that they needed adequate information, and it was largely because they felt the information to be lacking that the management of chronic conditions was troubled in so many cases.

References

[1] Davie, R., Butler, N. and Goldstein, H. (1972), *From Birth to Seven: the Second Report of the National Child Development Study (1958 Cohort).* London: Longman.

[2] *Scottish Health Statistics*, (1978), Edinburgh: HMSO.

[3] e.g. Lunn, J. E., Knowelden, J. and Roe, J. W. (1970), 'Patterns of respiratory illness in Sheffield junior school children: a follow-up study', *Brit. J. Prev. Soc. Med.*, **23**, 223.
Leeder, S. R., Corkhill, R. T., Wysock, M. J., Holland, W. W. and Colley, J. R. T. (1976), 'Influence of personal and family factors on ventilatory function of children', *Brit. J. Prev. Soc. Med.*, **30**, 219.
Miller, F. J. W., Court, S. D. M., Knox, E. G. and Brandon, S. (1974), *The School Years in Newcastle-on-Tyne*, London: Oxford University Press.
Douglas, J. W. B., Kiernan, K. E. and Wadsworth, M. E. J. (1977), 'A longitudinal study of health and behaviour', *Proc. Roy. Soc. Med.*, **70**, 530.
McKeown, T. and Record, R. G. (1976), 'Relationship between childhood infections and measured intelligence', *Brit. J. Prev. Soc. Med.*, **30**, 101.

[4] e.g. Oppé, T. E. (1967), 'Risk registers for babies', *Devel. Med. Child. Neurol.*, **9**, 13.
Walker, R. G. (1967), *An Assessment of the Current Status of the 'At Risk' Register*, Scottish Health Services Studies, no. 4, Edinburgh: Scottish Home and Health Department.
Alberman, E. D. and Goldstein, H. (1970), 'The "At Risk" register, a statistical evaluation', *Brit. J. Prev. Soc. Med.*, **24**, 129.
Wadsworth, M. E. J. and Morris, S. (1978), 'Assessing chances of hospital admission in pre-school children', *Arch. Dis. Childh.*, **53**, 159.

8 Accidents and Safety

Accidents have been selected as a special topic for consideration because accidental injury is a very important part of childhood mortality, and is the cause with the steepest gradient by social class. In 1970–72, mortality ratios for accidental death in children 1–14 years were four times as great in social class V as in social class I, and for deaths from falls, fire and drowning were ten times as great.[1]

Morbidity from accidents is, of course, more difficult to quantify. The major longitudinal studies of child health have shown considerable differences in the rates ascertained. Two of the early studies reported that 24.1 per cent of all the children studied had been accidentally injured by age 5,[2] and that every child had experienced about one accident by age 5.[3] Not only are these now some time ago, but the definition of 'accident' must remain problematic. Several studies have examined rates of accidents resulting in hospitalisation or attending hospital accident and emergency departments: an investigation by the Central Health Services Council[4] in 1960 produced rates of all children attending accident and emergency departments of 2.1/1000 for ages 0–4, and 2.3/1000 for ages 5–14. In the National Child Development Survey 3.56 per cent of children had been admitted to hospital for a road accident by 7 years, 10.02 per cent for a home accident, and 9.18 per cent for other accidents.[5]

There are, of course, problems about what is to be called an 'accident'. Simply counting everything that was reported to us, the number and age-distribution of incidents is shown in Table 8.1.

There is little difference between boys and girls in our sample. These are expressed as rates per year, of any accident, in Table 8.2.

Table 8.1   Accidents by sex and age

| | Age, years | | | | | | | |
| | 0–2 | | 3–5 | | 6–11 | | All children | |
	M	F	M	F	M	F	M	F
Number of accidents								
during 6 months survey	16	15	18	15	8	10	42	40
(Number of children at risk)	(20)	(22)	(28)	(21)	(21)	(27)	(69)	(70)

Table 8.2 *Rates of accident, child per year*

| | Rate | |
	M	F
Children 0–2	1.6	1.4
3–5	1.3	1.4
6–11	0.8	0.7
All children	1.2	1.1

These are obviously much higher than usually reported. However, we are considering many different types of accident, from trivial falls and bumps to injuries requiring hospitalisation: simply, these are the incidents the mothers reported to us when we inquired 'any accidents during the month?' Indeed, there were a few occasions on which a young child itself insisted on reporting a 'dreadful accident' when it was not clear that the mother would have thought it worth mentioning.

We probably have a complete and accurate record of all accidents which were taken for professional attention. Minor accidents are more problematic, since they depend so much on the mothers' perception of what should be reported. For the most part, these can be ignored (though very frequent minor injuries may be of interest).

Considering, therefore, only the more serious accidents, numbering 38, the nature of the accident, the place where it occurred, and the place where the child was treated are shown in Table 8.3.

Some accidents are, of course, inevitable where children are concerned, and we have no way of knowing whether this frequency of (more serious) accidents is any higher than 'normal'. The rate of 23/139 or 170/1000 children treated in hospital for accidental injury during 6 months is certainly higher than the figures already quoted, though this may be affected by the mothers' preference (to be discussed later) for presentation at the hospital.

This is only a six-months' record. In the children's medical history, and in the accounts given by the mothers of past health history, there were many serious or distressing injuries, but an exact description of these is not legitimate since we cannot be sure that the information is complete. Considering only hospital-treated injuries (which we are very likely to know about) comparatively few of the children had escaped, as shown in Table 8.4.

These figures also seem to represent a worse history of accidents than that which is usually reported.

Table 8.3 Circumstances of accidents occurring during the survey

	Number
Place of accident	
Inside house	13
Lobby, stairs and landing of tenement	4
Immediate vicinity of home—garden, playground, 'backie'	15
Public road	2
School	1
Other public place	3
Nature of accident	
Fall	12
Burn	3
Poisoning	2
Choking	1
Cut on glass	6
Things thrown, attack by other child	4
Caught in door	3
Bicycle accident	2
Foreign body in nose	1
Spade through toe	1
Dog bite	3
Treatment for accident	
Hospital inpatient	6
Hospital accident and emergency department	18
General practitioner called to home	1
Taken to general practitioner surgery	6
Dentist	2
Taken to child health clinic	1
No professional treatment	4

Table 8.4 History of hospital-treated injury

	Per cent who had never been treated in hospital for injury	(N = 100%)
Boys now aged:		
7 and over	0	(13)
5 and over	10	(30)
3 and over	20	(49)
Girls now aged:		
7 and over	19	(21)
5 and over	25	(32)
3 and over	27	(48)

The Causes of Accidents

All but 2 of the 13 accidents within the home were to toddlers of 3 years or less, and for the most part could be ascribed to the normal dangers associated with learning to walk, and climb, and explore the immediate environment. 'Unnecessary' dangers—unguarded fires, accessible poisons, untrained dogs, unsafe kitchens—must also be noted, but it would be unreasonable to suggest that any home can be made absolutely proof against a small child's ingenuity and curiosity. Typical accidents were a child playing on a chair, who fell and broke an arm; an infant, left playing on the floor while his mother was in the bathroom, who was severely attacked by a puppy; a three year old who ate contraceptive pills which she found in her mother's handbag; a six year old who stumbled against a table and knocked a pot of scalding tea over herself. There was no particular pattern apparent in these accidents, and very few occurred in the kitchen.

A greater proportion of accidents happened outside the home, but in its immediate environment. The majority of our families lived in tenement flats, in blocks between two and perhaps six storeys high, with communal stone staircases and landings and heavy doors on the ground floor at back and front. At the back there would be a communal 'green'—a misnomer in some cases for a bare, muddy area of ground—often unfenced and usually giving access to the road at the front. It was in these surroundings that most accidents occurred, rather than among the minority of families with their own gardens or among those living in tower-blocks. There were some accidents in the immediate environment of houses, frequently on the stone steps leading to the front door. Tower-blocks were considered by the mothers to be equally as bad an environment as tenements for young children, if not worse, and were felt to be full of dangers—high balconies, lifts that were attractive to play in, car-parks outside. However, small children living on, say, an 18th floor would never be allowed out on their own, so the dangers were not, in our sample, translated into any actual accidents.

It was our judgement that the environment of the tenement flats in the poorer council housing estates presented an unjustifiable degree of danger to the children, and it was only surprising that there were not more accidents. The stone staircases might be steep, uncarpeted, or with ragged carpets roughly stuck down. The children were usually not encouraged to play in lobbies, but in one block we observed: 'Ground-floor tenants evicted, four cats living there, Corporation clearing the rubbish, windows broken, lobby strewn with rubbish, children playing in it'. The heavy doors giving access to the outside might be permanently kept open, or might bang to and fro in the wind. The back greens, in the worst areas, were strewn with rusty metal and broken glass and frequented by roaming dogs. Some areas were fenced, but in those with the worst reputation all fences, front and back, had been removed to facilitate maintenance. The tenements might line major dual-carriage-ways, or face roads on which there was heavy suburban traffic. At least one of the roads on which our families lived was a well-known rush-hour diversion for motorists trying to avoid a major junction, though the tenants managed during the period of our survey to have it closed at one end so that this traffic was stopped. At the back of one of the housing estates there was a railway, with inadequate and broken fencing, onto which a deaf three-year-old child, the neighbour and nephew of one of our families, strayed and was killed during the survey period. Only at that point was an adequate fence provided.

To these physical dangers must be added the social dangers perceived by many of our mothers in the worst estates: older children who might throw bottles, neighbours whom they felt to be rough, disreputable, or 'strangers' of various sorts, deliberately housed in the most run-down areas. In one of the poorest estates where we had sample families, there was a case of child abduction and torture during the survey period which crystallised the fears of the mothers living nearby. The atmosphere of distrust amongst which many families had to live was vividly evoked by one mother, explaining her worries about her epileptic six year old 'going away with strangers':

> Once my father disguised himself and she went away with him. He warned me that I'd have to watch her. And there had been someone hanging around the school. Because of this their granda went to collect them one day and the police followed him all the way here. I managed to clear him, but the police took a bit of convincing!(M2)

There might, of course, be playgrounds provided for children (though one mother described how parents themselves had constructed a playground, only to have it 'chopped down for firewood' by neighbours) but reaching them would probably involve crossing busy roads. Commonly, children would play in carparks or on small areas of grass or shrubbery adjoining the road. M2, living in one of these areas, where the fences in front of the house had all been knocked down, described how her two year old had been found sitting in the road with cars all around, and said of her epileptic six year old:

> She will run out to meet her dad coming home. One day she stood

in the middle of the road when she saw her dad coming. You see, she's close to her dad, he spoils her because she takes the fits and has so many accidents.

Many mothers were eloquent about their fears for their children:

You either bring them up free to run about the streets when they're young or you don't. I couldnae dee it.(M12)
You don't let a kid of 2 or 3 out to play on its own—not around here, anyway. Maybe in the garden of a private house ... If you think anything of your kids you don't let them out to play here.(M13)
They say you can let them out when they're five, but I don't think I would do it. Not here.(M10)
It's too near the railway to let them outside to play. They would wander off.(M9)
If they play at the back the man downstairs often shoos them away because he rises early in the morning and sleeps in the afternoon. Then they'll go somewhere else and get into trouble there.(M1)

The problem about these tenements was that they fell between stools. It was not *impossible* to allow small children out, as it was in tower-blocks: the mother might feel that, as long as they were within the building or in the 'backie' she was not far away; she could 'keep an eye on them' from windows or by running down the stairs. Many mothers insisted that they *always* 'kept an eye' on the children: M55, for instance, talked obsessively of the safety of her two- and three-year-old children, and said 'When they go out the backie I sit on the step always. Sometimes I sit there and freeze.' The relationship between such statements and the mother's observed behaviour remains to be discussed. It may be noted, however, that the environment made it likely that children would very often be out of the sight of a mother three or four floors above the ground. Similarly, infants left in the house would be out of the hearing of a mother who had gone down to hang out her washing or dispose of rubbish, or who had 'just popped in' to a neighbour.

The Mothers' Behaviour
Safety within the home was a topic greatly stressed by health visitors. Typically, their criticisms involved unguarded fires, drugs left lying around, small children permitted to be up and playing when the parents were still in bed or left alone briefly while the mother was at a neighbour's or out shopping, snapping puppies, children seen hanging out of windows or playing on balconies, dangerous objects such as tacks and nails on the floor, pans within reach on cookers. We did observe many unguarded coal fires in homes where there

were toddlers, and many of our families had to rely for heating upon
electric fires with integral guards, certainly not proof against small
children. We also observed such things as children climbing behind
fire-guards, a three year old playing with electric sockets with wet
hands, or a two year old pushing keys into electric sockets. The
children seemed on the whole to survive without harm, however, and
not many of the accidents which occurred during the six months
could be ascribed to carelessness on the mother's part. There were no
accidents within the home which were caused by faulty equipment or
unguarded fires.

There was no association of a greater frequency of accidents with
the index of greater 'disadvantage'. Accidents were not more likely
for a child in overcrowded housing, or in families with economic
problems, or families where there was conflict. There was not, in our
sample, any association with a working mother. Certain problems
were presented to *all* our mothers. At what age should a child be
allowed out to play, either on its own or accompanied by older
children? For those with private gardens, or those high in tower-
blocks, this might not be an issue. For the rest, it was a common subject of discussion. A few mothers appeared to keep to very strict
rules for children under 5, but in many other cases though the
mother told us that a two or three year old was never allowed out
alone, we soon observed that this was not true. Should children of 5
and over go to school or to the shops by themselves? Most mothers
agreed that they would expect to, as most children did:

> Three weeks after he started school A. went on his own and my
> mother was furious. She said 'I took you up to the school till you
> were 7.' But I just said they have to learn sometime, and I've never
> seen kids more careful when they're crossing the road.(M5)

The fact that the mothers' accounts and their observed practice were
inconsistent did not necessarily mean that they were deliberately
trying to mislead us. They described what they would like to do, but
often found impossible. M2 described how the door had to be kept
locked to prevent her two year old from wandering away—but in
fact the child got bored and cried to be out, and was seen to play outside by a busy road. The two-year-old child of M14 was said to play
in the fenced back ground, with the gate tied, but he was observed in
the front with access to the road. M14 said:

> I shouldn't be in a house like this with four kids. They need their
> freedom. I don't like them playing outside on their own but I can't
> be with them if I've work to do in the house.

There were other practical problems: working mothers whose chil-

dren had to go to 'gran's' or to a neighbour after school, mothers who
baulked at dragging several small children on a quick trip to a shop,
mothers with infants who could not be left and toddlers who would
not stay in. It may be noted that quite a high proportion of the
accidents occurred when someone other than the mother was in
formal charge of the child.

Also, the real practices of the mother varied from child to child,
since each was an individual:

> C. had no common sense, I couldn't let her out before she was 5.
> But B. [deaf handicapped boy] could be left out to play from 1½, I
> knew he had a lot of common sense, he never got lost, he could
> find his way home after being anywhere once.(M53)
> F. was never out of the garden before 4. But M. has been in and
> out since he was 3.(M62)

In summary, and judging both by the history of hospitalised
accidents to the children in the past, and all the accidents recorded
during the survey, we would categorise 10 families as especially
accident-prone. These were families where every child had been
hospitalised for an accident, and where there was an average of at
least one accident per child in the family during the survey. Seven of
the families were living in very poor environments, but they have
little else in common: they do not, conspicuously, include the disturbed families or those where the mothers appeared to be most care-
less. Our conclusion has to be that only the environment is indicted.

Service-Use for Accidents
The mothers' service-use for accidents was relatively untroubled.
There were few occasions when they had difficulty in deciding
whether an injury merited treatment, and even if in doubt about its
seriousness, the majority of parents had no hesitation in taking the
child at once to the children's hospital. When M70's child caught the
tip of a finger in a door she said:

> I got a taxi and went straight up to the Sick Kids. That's what I'd
> always do—no messing about. I even picked up the little bit of
> finger and took it with me!

Accounts of the children's reception at the emergency department of
the hospital were, with only a single exception, enthusiastic. 'No
waiting', 'They were really nice', 'He couldn't have had better
attention' were the sorts of comments repeated many times. Even if
the definition of an 'emergency' was a little elastic, the parents were
not criticised: one night when a child started screaming, and the side
of his face was seen to be swollen, he was taken at once to the

hospital and mumps was diagnosed:

> I think they wanted us away quickly in case we spread it around, but she was pleasant enough. We went because it was so sudden. But you're never made to feel you're wasting their time.(M24)

As Table 8.3 showed, few accidents were taken to the general practitioner, though on one or two occasions he was telephoned and advised the parents to go straight to the hospital. One mother expressed the common principle clearly:

> If it's an accident, I'd never think of the doctor, I'd go straight to the hospital. They're very good, you don't have to wait. Anything like that, that's needing X-rays, all the doctor can say is this is needing the hospital. If they're ill, it's the doctor, if it's an accident, it's the hospital—I suppose that's my rule.(M53)

Since accidents were unlikely to happen conveniently during surgery hours, seeking attention from a general practitioner meant calling him to the house. This mothers were reluctant to do, if they were not sure that the injury was serious: to take the child to the hospital seemed not only easier but less of an imposition upon the services.

There were only two potential problems for our mothers concerning their use of emergency services. The first involved the practicalities of getting there, if a husband or a friendly neighbour with a car was not available. Several times, husbands were called home from work. Otherwise, taxis were commonly used (most mothers did not see the ambulance service as one which they could set in operation, although ambulances were called in several cases of convulsions) but there might be difficulties in finding a neighbour with a phone, or an unvandalised public phone, in order to call a taxi. The infant son of M27 pulled a cup of scalding coffee upon himself while the mother was collecting another child from school, and a friend who was 'watching' him took no steps until the mother returned. She then phoned for a taxi, but it took three-quarters of an hour to arrive. Eventually the child was admitted as an inpatient.

The same infant was admitted after having been attacked by a puppy, and the mother's account of her reception raises the second problem concerning the use of the emergency service—the occasional fear of accusations of lack of care or even 'non-accidental injury':

> I didn't like the questions they asked me, but I suppose they have to do it. It was the same thing over and over again. Where was I at the time? Had the dog ever done that to the others?

And, on the occasion of the scalding:

They make you feel as if you took the cup of coffee and throwed it on top of him!

Another woman said, of the waiting-room she was sent to:

> ... I thought it was where they see about cruelty. I was sitting with a bunch of people who looked as though they would beat up their kids. But it was just to see about some procedure ... (M24)

There was in fact one family in our sample where there was an unequivocal record of 'battering' (by the husband) in the child's record, and three others where the possibility had, in the past, been raised. These families were obviously most at risk of being treated with suspicion, but the fears about a child's injury being misinterpreted which were generally expressed, even by the most careful and loving of mothers, were a sad commentary on the way which mothers in this social group thought they might be stigmatised:

> When we came back from the hospital everyone in the bus was staring, a baby like that with a great plaster on her arm, and then it dawned on me they might think she'd been battered.(M66)
> There was one time ... I went up (to the clinic) with the three of them and J. had blacked his eye, he hurt it on the window sill, I think it was. And the doctor had a look at it, and he says 'How is his eye all black and blue ... how did it happen?' It was sort of first degree, ken, I felt as though, gee, he maybe thinks I belt him or something! ... And then I was up with C., she was 6 months, I was up to get the injection, and when he took her she'd a red mark. 'And what's this on this baby's heid?' And I says, it's the shape o' the bobble on her hat, if you look, I said, it's off her hat, like, pressing in. And I says, what do you think I was doing, beating the kids up or something?(M1)

On this occasion the clinic personnel were aware that the mother was upset by the doctor's questioning, and M1 recounted a long story of her conversation with them:

> The nurse says, 'Well, dinna worry yourself, it's just that there is an awful lot of it going on, and they're just making sure about it, ken?' And I says, Oh aye, but I felt really horrible about it ... But they ken bruises that's been done wi' falling and bruises that's been done wi' hitting. So that put me right off going back to the clinics.(M1)

One health visitor suggested to us that obvious suspicions of carelessness or non-accidental injury might have the unfortunate effect of making a mother 'think twice about taking a child to the hospital' because she had been made to feel guilty. There might be some support for this in M1's account. We have no evidence from her behaviour, however, or that of any other mother, that these fears influenced in any way their generally enthusiastic use of the emergency service.

References

[1] Macfarlane, A. and Fox, J. (1978), 'Child deaths from accident and violence', *Population Trends*, **12**, London: HMSO.

[2] Douglas, J. W. B. and Blomfield, J. M. (1958), *Children under Five*. The results of a National Survey made by a Joint Committee of the Institute of Child Health, the Society of Medical Officers of Health and the Population Investigation Committee, London: Allen and Unwin.

[3] Miller, F. J. W., Court, S. D. M., Walton, W. S. and Knox, E. G. (1960), *Growing up in Newcastle-on-Tyne*, London: Oxford Univ. Press for the Nuffield Foundation.

[4] Central Health Services Council, Standing Medical Advisory Committee (1962), *Accident and Emergency Services*, London: HMSO.

[5] Davie, R., Butler, N. and Goldstein, H. (1972), *From Birth to Seven: the Second Report of the National Child Development Study (1958 Cohort)*. London: Longman.

9 Dental Care

Most of the British literature on dental care indicates that parents in the lowest social classes put a rather low value on the preservation of teeth. Many studies have shown that non-manual families in various areas of Britain tend to be better informed and more favourable towards preventive care, which may still be viewed as a luxury by some manual families.[1] Of the children in the National Child Development Survey over seven years, 83.31 per cent of children in social class I families had ever attended a dentist, dental clinic or orthodontist, with the proportion falling regularly with social class to 67.57 per cent in social class V. In social class I families 15.56 per cent of children had no missing, filled or carious teeth, falling to 9.97 per cent in social class IV and 11.18 per cent in social class V. However, particularly relevant to our survey, the variation by area was found to be greater than the variation by class, ranging from 18.77 per cent of children with no missing, filled or carious teeth in the Eastern area to only 6.45 per cent in Scotland.[2]

Similar class and regional differences were found in an OPCS study of five year olds.[3] Forty per cent of children in social class IV and V had never seen a dentist, 32 per cent in social class III manual and 18 per cent in social class I, II and III non-manual combined. The most remarkable difference between the classes, however, was in the treatment received. Children from non-manual classes were much more likely to have attended at three years of age or earlier, and to have attended without receiving any treatment. Children from social class IV and V were more likely to have had extractions and less likely to have had fillings.[3]

There is no doubt that our sample of mothers tended to give low priority to dental care both for themselves and their children. For those aged three and over (97 children), in the 579 'child-months' of the six-months' survey there were 111 months with reported dental problems, i.e. about one month in five. (This probably represents considerable under-reporting, as many mothers told us that their children had decayed teeth only at the end of the study, although this had probably been the case throughout. Undoubtedly the children's dental health was worse than these figures show.) Of these symptoms

74, or 67 per cent, were not attended to during that month. Thirty children aged three and over, approximately 30 per cent of those at risk, had never been to a dentist except in an emergency. Only four children appeared to have reached five years of age with no dental decay or treatment, i.e. 6.45 per cent of those aged five and over. This is a very similar figure to that reported in the NCDS for Scotland. We know that several of the children had second teeth filled or removed.

The *structure* of dental services in the City is of course relevant. All primary school and local authority nursery school children have their teeth checked periodically by a school dentist; if treatment is believed to be necessary a card is sent to the parents, who are also asked to select school or 'private' care for their child. If the former is chosen, an appointment is made for the child to attend the nearest health clinic which accommodates school dental facilities; if the latter course is selected, it is the responsibility of parents to decide where the child is treated, if at all. For the whole Region in which the City is situated, routine statistics[4] demonstrate that in fact a high proportion of all school children—about 70 per cent—receive dental examinations at school. This may be compared with a figure of about 44 per cent for Scotland as a whole. The proportion who are then found to have defects, about 55 per cent of those examined, is not far from the Scottish average. The proportion of those with defects who accept treatment, however, is only about one-third, and is consistently the lowest among Scottish Health Boards. The Region (though not necessarily, of course, the City) also compares poorly with others in the availability of dental surgeons in primary care (a rate, in 1978, of 20.9 per 100,000 population, compared with an average for all Scotland of 23.6).

Mothers' Dental Health

As the literature shows, the dental care of children is often associated with their mothers' dental status. Although we collected little information about the dental care practised by the older generation—the grandmothers—it is clear that the young women's teeth had been neglected in childhood. Indeed, according to the available 1950–53 data on part of our sample at the age of five, only a tiny minority had been taken to the dentist for preventive care; most of the girls were recorded as having 'terrible teeth', in many cases 'deformed and carious', and had attended a dentist for extractions only, if at all.

Now, only 18 (31 per cent) of the mothers made regular non-emergency visits to a dentist (at least once a year); generally, but not invariably, these were the families where the children also attended on a regular basis. At least 11 (19 per cent) either had a considerable number of false teeth or were completely edentulous; generally their teeth had been extracted in their late teens and early twenties:

> I've got false teeth because I didn't look after my teeth. Once I'd left school and started taking a pride in my appearance, it was too late.(M7)

Several of the women decided to have all their teeth extracted whilst pregnant or before their children were a year old, because the procedure was free, and never regretted it.

Most of the remaining women delayed seeking treatment for themselves until the last possible moment. M1 reported that she suffered 'in agony' for days until crushing analgesic tablets against the tooth inflamed her mouth. Other mothers said:

> No, I'm afraid I don't go to the dentist very much . . . I went to my dentist and I said, 'My teeth are falling to bits', I said, 'Take out the ones that are needing attention', I says, 'I'm not coming in for any fillings' I told him, 'I'm not having any fillings, just take out the ones that need out.' So that's what I got, and I've never been back since.(M8)
> I remember going when I was 15. I had to have my mum with me. I sat their shakin' all over. I'll keep away from dentists if I can. I'd rather have another baby than have a tooth out.(M51)
> I'm a coward with the dentist—I'll wait till my teeth a' fa' oot an' then I'll start an' complain aboot it.(M36)

A considerable number of the mothers claimed to have been 'put off for life by the school dentist'.

Such poor dental health and care in this group of mothers did not inevitably mean that their children's teeth were completely neglected, although it was among these families that the worst care occurred. Many women, however, said that they had learnt their lesson the hard way and were reluctant for their children to suffer to the same extent:

> I'd like them to look after their teeth. I think you learn from yourself.(M3)
> I dinna want them to end up like me.(M9)
> *My* mother didn't make me go, but I make *mine* go.(M23 and M27)

and others similarly made it clear that fear of the dentist was one attitude that could be passed on through the generations:

> It's the mothers saying 'Oh, I'm feart' and the kids is sittin' listenin' to you sayin' that.(M70)

Preventive Care for the Children

Most of the mothers admitted some responsibility for their children's poor teeth very freely:

> It's wi' eatin' too much sweeties.(M16)
> I spoiled their teeth by using a dummy to comfort them.(M19)

Only a few women claimed that they encouraged their family to eat fruit and crisps rather than sugar foods.

One mother had her eight-year-old daughter's teeth coated with fluoride every two months, for which she paid, and another seriously considered this measure for her daughter. Three others claimed to give their children fluoride drops or tablets, but in one case this was probably only occasional. Another mother had once given her son fluoride, but now felt that at two and a half 'he's probably too old'; this mother, generally keen on preventive care, did not envisage giving fluoride to her baby:

> C. didn't have them and his teeth are perfect. The clinic said he had perfect teeth. They didn't have these things before and kids did all right. I think they are maybe over-protected now. C. cleans his teeth, eats fruit and toast, so his teeth should be all right. Mind you, some babies don't get the right food and the early years matter for teeth.(M37)

Our findings concerning tooth brushing can only be approximate; those mothers who discussed the matter tended to give 'acceptable' replies, e.g. one single-handed parent claimed that her children cleaned their teeth regularly, but their brushes were kept at her boyfriend's flat, which she visited only at weekends. About half of the families appeared to have a regular tooth brushing routine for the children. Some of the women's comments on the subject provide illustrations of their general attitude.

> They'll decide to clean their teeth at right awkward times—like, last thing at night when they're awa' to their beds—and I give them into trouble. Then I say 'I shouldnae dae that'—and everybody I've spoken to, their kids are the same, they never keep to a sort of routine of cleaning.(M1)
> [Daughter] . . . [who has had second teeth extracted] doesn't look after them either—at night she sometimes says she has done them and she hasn't. But you can't follow an 11 year old everywhere.(M12)
> The last health visitor tried to teach me to clean [one-year-old daughter's] teeth with a cotton bud. She only had about 3 teeth. I just said 'Oh yes' and leave them to do it in their own time.(M30)

This last mother had tried to force her children to brush their teeth and found this ineffective:

I said, well, if they've got bad teeth, and they don't do it, it's their own fault.(M30)

and this was echoed by M31:

I don't press him [three-year-old son] too much. He's a bit young to get involved with his teeth.

Data on preventive visits to the dentist are difficult to quantify, because of the routine checks of all primary and nursery school children. However, roughly one third of the mothers with children for whom regular checks might be appropriate (children aged three and over) either took no initiative for preventive visits if their child was not attending school, said that they took their children regularly but did not do so during the six months, or ignored cards from school suggesting that the child visit a dentist. Rather, these mothers used the dental services, if at all, purely for emergency purposes when severe toothache occurred. They believed that preventive care was rather pointless for milk teeth—'not unless they have toothache', or 'not unless it was necessary'.

Roughly another third relied entirely on the school or nursery dental screening to detect problems. Seventeen women, on the other hand, tried to ensure that their children attended their 'own' dentist at least six-monthly (occasionally every three or four months) in addition to the school screening, or made preventive visits to the school dentist on their own initiative, frequently commencing at the age of three. One three year old was taken 'to get used to it . . . so that if he ever needed treatment he would ken a dentist's chair' (M29). M70 tried to encourage her family to look on the visits to the dentist as 'fun' and genuinely attempted to ensure regular visits, saying 'I dinna want it to come to an emergency'. Others among this group of mothers made comments such as:

I don't see why my kids should be scared. It's not a bad thing, it's a good thing for them.(M30)
My mother drilled it into me to go to the dentist. We try to do the same with F.(M32)

Curative Services
We have noted that 67 per cent of dental symptoms were not attended to in the month in which they occurred. Although several of the mothers commented that they would hate to see their children in pain—'there's no need to suffer from toothache' (M61)—one third of the women consistently ignored decay and/or suffering, believing that symptoms occurring between school checks somehow did not count, ignored cards sent from school, or regularly forgot appoint-

ments and did not make fresh ones:

> But it's just a carry on. She'll be munching a sweet and half an
> hour after she'll complain of her teeth. But she's the first one to go
> for the sweets.(M2)

Some examples of neglect recorded during the six-months' survey
follow: because of chest trouble the six-year-old son of M30 did not
keep an appointment for the extraction of a tooth with an abscess at
the root; M30 waited *six months* before making another appointment with her own dentist. The two- and three-year-old children of
M55 both suffered from toothache, and one had a visible abscess;
they were dosed with Junior Aspirin and never taken to the dentist:

> Well, *I* would if they're suffering, but he [husband] doesn't believe
> in it. He says if the dentist gets to them young, their second teeth
> suffer.(M55)

The two year old had screamed out one day while eating a meal:

> My husband was sure she'd broken a tooth but we couldn't see
> anything and she wouldn't stop screaming. Then he said 'I'll give
> her some ice-cream that'll stop it.' And it did—and she hasn't
> complained since.(M55)

All the child's front teeth remained broken and decayed, but the
mother placed the responsibility on her husband: 'He says, "Leave
it, they'll fall out soon."' Another mother said, of her seven year
old:

> He needs to go now—he's got holes round the bottom of his teeth
> at the gums. He'll have to wait until after the holidays [by
> September she had not arranged this]. Someone told him that's
> called Polo holes. So I told him—no more Polos.(M71)

Although there were conflicting opinions on restorative work for
children's teeth, generally the women's views were unfavourable.
Only one mother considered changing her dentist because he refused
to fill the teeth of three- and six-year-old children, and gave this as a
reason or excuse for not attending. The most common reaction was
that of M40:

> He got one fillin' in the front an' that's the only een that's stayed
> in, the ither two came oot. They werenae even in a week. So to me
> it's a waste of time fillin' their teeth, they're just as well takin' the
> teeth oot there an' then.(M40)

Dental Services
In a large proportion of the sample there was an almost obsessive fear
and dislike (M6 referred to 'stigma') for the school dental services

and many absolutely refused to have their children treated by them:

> I don't believe in the school dentist. I went myself and I know
> what it's like—that was enough to put anyone off dentists.(M5)
> I once went with my cousin—she was in two seconds and had two
> teeth out. Her mouth couldn't have been frozen . . . That put me
> off the school dentist for life. It's bad enough getting kids to go to
> a dentist anyway.(M10)
> I wouldn't let them go to the school dentist. I'd get a dentist for
> them. I think they'd be more friendly with children. The school
> dentist is dealing with kids all the time, so he's not interest-
> ed.(M16)

On the other hand, most of the 17 mothers who *did* choose to have
their children treated regularly by the school dentist (or were forced
to because it was impossible to get any other) were fairly satisfied
with the service. If the child could be treated at the local health clinic
mothers with other young children found this extremly convenient.
These mothers admitted that dentists had changed:

> Some people say 'Oh, they'll go to my own dentist.' But I think the
> school dentist is dealing with children all the time and understands
> them better.(M12)
> Before there used to be a stigma against the school dentist. But it's
> been OK with [daughter] up till now.(M6)

Nevertheless, the majority of mothers would not dream of letting a
school dentist near their child (apart from routine screening) and
sought their own dentist (if any) as an ideal. However, this was often
fraught with difficulties, and in many cases led to symptoms being
neglected for long periods or the use of emergency services. A few of
the families had attended the same practice for years, were sent
regular appointment cards, and were happy with the services. But
practices regularly closed down or moved, some dentists became ill
or died, and many refused to take on more patients or began to take
private patients only. Even highly motivated mothers—and we have
seen that they were in the minority where dental care was concerned—became discouraged, confused and angry. Children with
raging toothache had to wait for as long as a week, even more, for an
appointment with their 'own' dentist, and mothers were often
reluctant to use the emergency service since they believed that they
were 'registered' with a practitioner.

Examples included M4, whose dentist gave up business and
reopened several times, refused to answer the phone, took appointments, yet was firmly shut when the child arrived. The other dentists
in the vicinity would not accept her children because she was not one
of their patients. Another mother wandered round several practices

seeking attention for her own 'raging toothache', but all were too busy and merely put her name on a list: 'I've got earache with it, and it's driving me up the wall.' (M25) Some mothers discovered that there were *no* dentists for miles around.

· The case of M70 sums up many of these problems. Her children had been accustomed to attending the dentist and she was highly motivated towards regular screening and treatment, as long as this did not involve the school facilities. However, she discovered that her regular dentist had given up business and when she attempted to have her three children checked by the two practices nearby, one was 'only taking emergency patients', the other 'not taking any more patients'. When her son, aged four, developed a gumboil, she tried to have him treated by the nearest practice as an emergency, but was refused. Her health visitor advised her to use a health centre several miles away, a problem for a single parent with three young children. She said:

> There aren't enough dentists. We should have as many dentists as doctors, in groups the same way.(M70)

Dental Care and 'Disadvantage'

We have demonstrated that the dental health and dental care of the children in our sample was poor, as commonly found in other surveys of these social classes. The relationship of dental care to the index of 'disadvantage' of the child's family is shown in Table 9.1.

Table 9.1 *Relationship of children's dental care to the index of 'disadvantage' of the family*

	Children three years and over who are in families characterised as	
	'Less disadvantaged'	*'More disadvantaged'*
Use of preventive services:		
None (except for school services for children 5 +)	22 (52%)	47 (85%)
Regular preventive checks by dentist	20 (48%)	8 (15%)
Use of dental treatment (during six-months' survey)		
Acute symptoms but no treatment	6 (14%)	23 (42%)
No apparent symptoms	27 (64%)	21 (38%)
Symptoms which were treated	9 (22%)	11 (20%)
(N = 100%)	(42)	(55)

It is clear that those children whose dental care was poor were those who were 'disadvantaged' in other ways, and that dental care bears a closer relationship to patterns of use of preventive measures, such as immunisation, than to the use of medical services for acute illnesses. Not only were the children in the 'more disadvantaged' families conspicuously less likely to have regular preventive checks (except for the school services), but they were also more likely to have experienced acute episodes of dental symptoms during the survey period. About one third of the children over three in the 'less disadvantaged' group experienced toothache or other symptoms during the six months, but nearly two-thirds of those in the 'more disadvantaged'. (There were also one or two children younger than three years, as has been noted.) These children were also much more likely to go without treatment.

References

[1] e.g. Dickson, S. (1968), 'Class attitudes to dental treatment', *Sociology*, **19**, 206

Beal, J. F. and James, P. M. C. (1970), 'Social differences in the dental conditions and dental needs of 5 year old children in four areas of the West Midlands', *Brit. Dent. J.*, **129**, 313.

Vorgan, W. I. (1970), 'Dental knowledge and attitudes: an investigation', *Brit. Dent. J.*, **128**, 481.

[2] Davie, R., Butler, N. and Goldstein, H. (1972), *From Birth to Seven: the Second Report of the National Child Development Study (1958 Cohort)*, London: Longman.

[3] Todd, J. E. (1975), *Children's Dental Health in England and Wales, 1973*, London: HMSO.

[4] *Scottish Health Statistics*, yearly, Edinburgh: HMSO.

10 Immunisation

We examined the patterns of immunisation among our sample in detail for several reasons. It is generally believed that in social classes IV and V the uptake of this preventive measure is lower than in other groups, with the result that children already at risk due to factors in their environment are felt to be exposed to further danger. In addition, doubts concerning the side effects of whooping-cough vaccine (and perhaps measles vaccine) have brought the topic into the arena of public debate. It is therefore of interest to study the attitudes and behaviour of our special group of mothers in the light of this controversy.

Other studies have tended to show that failure to immunise children, though it does demonstrate a clear social-class gradient, is particularly marked in groups defined as specially 'disadvantaged'. In the children of the National Child Development Survey at seven years, while only 1 per cent in social class I remained unprotected against polio, the figure was 10 per cent in social class V.[1] When the 6 per cent of the sample who were defined as 'disadvantaged' at 11 years were compared with the rest, however, they were found to be disproportionately the unimmunised, e.g. one seventh were not immunised against diphtheria.[2] A more recent cohort study, *Child Health and Education in the Seventies*,[3] has reported similar findings.

For our sample, the current pre-school immunisation programme consisted of a course of three injections of triple vaccine (diphtheria, tetanus and whooping cough) in conjunction with oral polio vaccine, recommended between the ages of roughly three months and ten months; measles vaccine at about one year; rounded off by a booster of diphtheria, tetanus and oral polio vaccine prior to commencing school. Recently mothers have been able to omit the whooping-cough component of the triple vaccine. In the past, for the older grandmothers, a more restricted programme was available, consisting of smallpox vaccination and diphtheria immunisation. Protection against polio and whooping cough (both by injection) was introduced at a later date, and this may have been available for the children of the younger grandmothers in our sample.

The Grandmothers

Nine of the 50 grandmothers (18 per cent) on whom we have data (from 1950–53 and/or from interviews) refused or ignored vaccination and/or immunisation for their children. We have no check on what they told us in the cases where the women were not in the 1950–53 sample, nor detailed information on any delays in obtaining the procedures, but where we have the earlier records the consistency of reporting over time is remarkable.

The negative influences on the women who refused immunisation are of interest. One was not immunised because her grandmother, with whom they lived, disapproved; as a consequence she claimed that she 'took the drawback' with whooping cough which 'left a weakness in the chest' responsible for her subsequent ill health. Similarly, another grandmother was fully supported by *her* mother in not taking her children for immunisation:

> We had a health visitor, an' she wis een o' them kind—that just thought she kent a' thing—but once they went to the school they got a' their needles, cos I just telt them straight oot that I didnae bother wi' them. If she hidnae been persistent, I probably would have got them done. But I mean, I could just have phoned the doctor and gotten them done. Cos, well, touch wood, there's nuthin' happened to my three.(G13)

Another woman claimed that a 'dirty needle' had been used when *her* mother had some of her children vaccinated; as a result neither she nor her daughter had received protection:

> So consequently *I* never got mine done. You see? It's goin' in—runs in [the family].(G22)

Other grandmothers said that they had refused vaccination for their children for other reasons:

> And then when I had the boy they said they wouldn't do it until he was a year old and I says well, no way was I goin' to get it done, because he was such a boisterous boy that the least knock he would give himself he would have knocked the scab right off. And he would really have made an awful mess of his arm. I said, well, if they can't do it at 6 weeks, why should I let them do it at a year in *their* time . . . It's my child, it should be me that says when he gets the needle and when he doesn't.(G30)

or offered no explanation at all:

> I think they got them a' done when they went to the school. Because I never bothered wi' clinics or onything. I dinna think ony o' them's vaccinated either.(G31)

However, the majority of grandmothers expressed themselves as being very much in favour of immunisation now, and many talked in a knowledgeable way about the controversy regarding whooping-cough or measles vaccines.

Immunisation Records of the Sample Children

In the young families, eight children in six families had received no triple or polio immunisation before attending school at five, or (if they were younger) it was clear that they were unlikely to. Eighteen children in 13 families were immunised very late or had an incomplete record by the age of five. As shown in Table 10.1, there were small numbers of other children whose immunisation had been medically advised against, or who were at the present time late for medical reasons. Also, four mothers had refused measles vaccine for nine children, and ten mothers had refused whooping-cough vaccine for 12 children.

It may be noted that these figures are, in fact, slightly above the averages (for all social classes) for Scotland as a whole.[4] In 1978, considering children of five years old, 77.6 per cent had received the basic immunisations. Our children unimmunised against measles and whooping cough were a much smaller proportion than the unimmunised in Scotland among five year olds in 1978 (30.8 per cent and 48.5 per cent respectively) though the spread of ages in this

Table 10.1   Immunisation: records of the children

	Number of children	
No triple or polio by age 5 (or no likelihood of child under 5)	8	
Late or incomplete record, without health reasons	18	
Late (child still an infant) because mother or child was ill	3	
Incomplete on medical advice	6	
All children with late or incomplete records, who may be counted more than once above (measles and whooping cough excluded)	29	(20.9%)
Children with complete records (measles and whooping cough not taken into account)	110	(79.1%)
Measles vaccine refused	9	
Whooping-cough vaccine refused	12	
Children with complete records (including measles and whooping cough)	97	(69.8%)
(N = 100%)	(139)	

sample, in relation to the timing of debates about these vaccines, makes the comparison problematic.

Since mothers might, of course, be likely to neglect immunisation or refuse one component for more than one of their children, the proportion of *families* where every child was completely immunised—52 per cent of all families (see Table 10.2)—was less than the proportion of children with complete records—70 per cent of all children.

Table 10.2   Mothers' immunisation practices

	Number of children
One or more children none, late or incomplete	16 (28%)
One or more children with deliberate delays or omissions (only)	12 (21%)
All children complete	30 (52%)
(N = 100%)	(58)

It was particularly notable that, as Table 10.3 shows, the children with incomplete records *without* medical reasons or deliberate choice were all, with one exception, in the 'more disadvantaged' group of families. Some women in each group had deliberately chosen to omit part of the programme, but in the 'more' disadvantaged there was a greater likelihood of other parts of the programme being late or omitted as well, with no medical or conscientious grounds.

Table 10.3   Relationship of children's immunisation record to index of 'disadvantage' of the family

	Children in families characterised as:	
	'Less disadvantaged'	'More disadvantaged'
None, late or incomplete	1	25 (32%)
Only delays or omissions for medical reasons or by choice	10 (16%)	6 (8%)
Complete	51 (82%)	46 (60%)
(N = 100%)	(62)	(77)

Achievement of completed immunisation programmes counted as 'success' for many health visitors, and they devoted much time to persuasion of the wary and reminding of the tardy: 'If the mother has the child immunised it's half the battle.' They said in interview that, although few families in their case-load neglected immunisation nowadays, the frustration caused by the few was great. Completed immunisation was almost proof of a 'caring' parent, and non-immunisation of the reverse.

However, the system for obtaining immunisation was sometimes rather confused. Some women preferred to have children done by their own GP, either during surgery hours or on special clinic days; others regularly used local authority doctors in health clinics, either because their own GP would not take on this task, or because the mothers found this more convenient; some mothers adopted a combination of methods for different children or for the same child. Because of this divided responsibility some health visitors, the guardians of the overall programme, often had little idea how it was progressing, although cards were kept at the various locations:

> We prefer them to have them done at the GP because we can't keep tabs on them otherwise.

As more health visitors became GP-attached, rather than area-based at local authority clinics, the confusion may have been reduced slightly. Nevertheless problems still arose when the health visitor was area-based and the mother said that the child had been immunised by her GP, or where the health visitor was GP-attached and the mother claimed that she used the clinic for immunisation.

Latecomers and Defaulters
The latecomers and persistent defaulters among the young mothers were very diverse in attitude and intention, although as a rule they were not opposed to immunisation in principle. Rather they found it difficult or unpleasant for various reasons to attend when health visitors considered it appropriate. (It is possible that a few of these children might not have been immunised at all, had it not been for this study, although we in no way indicated disapproval of non-immunisation; several 2 and 3 year olds were taken for the first time during the 6 months.)

Some of this group of mothers found the experience traumatic:

> I don't like the thought of taking her. I'm scared in case she jerks when I'm holding her. It's not that I'm really scared of injections myself. But when I was expecting and was getting an injection in the arm, the nurse's hand slipped and I was bruised the length of my arm—I wouldn't mind so much if someone else took her to be injected.(M10)

The father took the child during the study. Similarly M64 admitted that her child was 'late' because 'It turns me over seeing injections' and she wished her husband to accompany her, and his free time seldom coincided with clinic hours.

Many, like M19, found the clinic or surgery inconvenient or inaccessible with several small children; her local clinic had been closed down and during the study she defaulted many appointments at one further away, until the health visitor took her by car. The oldest boy was at school before he received his 'booster'. Therefore the location of clinics was an important factor, but there were few instances of health visitors providing transport, and only one mother, with four children, said that her GP had given immunisations at home.

The majority of latecomers claimed that the child suffered constant colds (very common as we have seen) and other minor morbidity:

> He's always had colds or dry skin when he was due to get done. When it's clear I can't manage to go, and when I can manage he has this dry skin.(M14)
> They won't look at him when he has a cold.(M21)
> I can't see her getting it done till the warmer weather.(M30)

However, very few mothers appeared to be concerned about this delay. The mother of one five year old who had large gaps in his record said:

> If he takes it, he takes it. Anyway, it doesn't stop them taking it. They just don't take it so bad.(M30)

Health visitors, frustrated by the delays (often related to defaulting in attendance at routine assessments also), referred to these mothers as 'lackadaisical' and 'apathetic', disregarding their excuses. 'You just have to keep at it—keep going back.'

Whooping-Cough and Measles Immunisations

For some mothers, it was the controversy over whooping-cough and measles immunisations which had confused the issue. This was a topic of considerable interest to most of the young mothers, though the level of knowledge of some seemed to be limited—'some baby died or something' (M28) or:

> No, it was the polio one there was all that fuss about, wasn't it. It could give you brain damage. But I wouldn't pay any attention to that—there's a lot of polio these days, it's best to be done.(M64)

A few heard about the controversy only when they attended for the child's first injection, and made spur-of-the-moment decisions:

> Well, it was actually the head health visitor that I saw when I got her first needle, an' she says to me 'Do you want the 2 or the 3?' I

says 'What do you mean, the 2 or the 3?' She says 'Are you
wantin' to leave out the whooping cough?' And I says 'Well, what
div [do] you advise?' She says 'Well, it's nae up to me, it's up to
yoursel'.' But I just got the three . . . I just made up my mind there
and then.(M40)

A considerable number were content to leave any decisions up to the
medical profession, so that the responsibility was taken out of their
hands:

When M. was born the programmes came on the TV about the
handicapped children. I thought it was a big chance to take, but
the doctor said it would be all right. But I mean, I wis only 19, and
at that age I dinna think you hae much o' an idea whit's right and
whit's wrang, so if the doctor says he can get it, you jist go ahead,
cos you feel that they ken a lot better than fit [what] you do.(M36)

Several others were fully aware of the debate, but after some thought
concluded that the benefits of full immunisation outweighed the
risks, since whooping cough appeared to be such a 'nasty' disease:

It's a risk you've got to take. I've seen a child really ill with
whooping cough, but it's a million to one risk of brain damage.
You've just got to cross your fingers and hope that everything goes
OK for them. If you bring a child into the world, you've got to
protect it. Not let it get every disease that's going. You might as
well make a good job of it.(M7)
The doctor asked me if I wanted whooping cough done with the
last one [child] [Why?] They say it can cause brain damage. [Did
the doctor mention it?] I know, watching TV, they've had it on
Nationwide. I often watch programmes like that.(M52)

She had the injection done because 'it hadn't done the others any
harm' and 'whooping cough can be nasty—the boy downstairs had it
and it didn't go away for three months'. Another mother said,
however:

But I had a lot of doubt with the baby about whooping cough—I'd
watched as much things on TV. I went and asked the doctor and
he said it's best to get it done. But afterwards I stood and watched
over him for a whole day, to see if there was anything wrong. [She
then saw a programme about the effects of the disease] So I was
glad that I'd had it done—it would kill him if he was ill like that at
his age.(M66)

Another small group of mothers made a considered decision to omit
the whooping-cough component of the triple vaccine, though several
expressed concern and confusion:

I wouldn't have the whooping-cough vaccine. It seems to me that the percentage of children that get brain damage from it and the percentage of babies that die from it is just about the same. It's six of one and half a dozen of the other . . . I don't know, I just—if it came to the fact that you were ha'in a straight choice, would you rather see your child dead or brain damaged, you know, useless for the rest of its life—I'm afraid I'd rather see my children dead. Nae that brain damaged children canna be happy in themselves, but you're goin' to get too old to look after them . . . I mean, they dinna ken everything about it. You keep hearing about it on the TV and they want children immunised, and then you hear about them expecting to get compensation for children damaged by the vaccine . . . (M8)

Another mother pondered at length, and discussed the problem with her husband and relatives before refusing the whooping-cough element:

They [at the clinic] didn't really advise me. I think there's been too much about it on TV . . . It's between the devil and deep blue sea—I think 3 months is a bit young. D. didn't get it done till 6 months. I think you need time to get to know the baby, what he's like. They ask if he has asthma and fits, but these are the sorts of things you wouldn't learn till later when he's spoon fed. [But she fervently believed in starting the other parts of immunisation] Because you hae to think of the other diseases, like polio and diphtheria.(M37)

Her decision against the whooping-cough vaccine was mainly based on the fact that her nephew was not given it:

. . . since he had taken twitching as a baby. They are first cousins, you're never sure. There's always something they find out.

In another family, the elder girl had not been given the whooping-cough injection:

. . . because she had jaundice and they wouldn't do her—I don't know why. Then I didn't want to chance it with her sister when there was that brain damage scare. [What did the doctor say?] He says we canna say get it done or don't get it done. But it's up to you. [So how did you decide?] I talked to my husband and he says 'If you're the least bit worried don't have it.' [The children thereafter contracted whooping cough, so the mother was asked, Are you sorry now?] No—they've been ill, but that's it over now. Brain damage you wouldn't get over.(M64)

There was also considerable fear of the measles vaccine, and a few mothers avoided it on a matter of principle. One woman's nephew had been advised by the doctor not to have it done, which planted the seeds of doubt in her mind:

There I was gaun [going] to get mine done, but I was expecting J. at the time—they advised me not to get it done because I was expecting—it could blind the baby or onything—then that just put me mair and mair against it. Cos there's aye that chance that it could happen tae the odd one.(M4)

These fears and controversies were frequently among the reasons mentioned by those mothers who had refused any immunisation at all for one or more of their children. Although she had had both her boys immunised one mother stopped visiting the health clinic with her six-month-old girl when the 'scare' was given press and television coverage, and she never returned. She did not realise that she could have the other components done, regretted her decision later when she imagined that her two year old had suffered whooping cough, and watched each cold with trepidation:

> They said that now if she got the whooping-cough one she would really go mental, so they're not giving it.

Another woman was decidedly confused about the matter and no health visitor appeared to have attempted to clarify the issue:

> I don't want those first needles, and they [clinic] won't have you unless you'll hae the needles. [Which ones?] Just the first ones, my husband won't have it. [And you agree?] Yes—it's the brain damage, they can give you brain damage. [Would you have the polio done, for instance?] Yes, I wouldn't mind that. [Have you asked the doctor to give you the ones you don't mind?] No, our doctor won't do them. It has to be the clinic, and I can't go there because they haven't had the first ones.(M55)

M16 refused any immunisation at all, associating every one with 'the scare'; however, there undoubtedly was no controversy about whooping cough when her five year old was a baby. Probably this mother delayed because:

> I don't like needles anyway...I dinna like the thought o' onybody stickin' a needle in my bairn.

However, later she found a 'better' reason:

> What really put me off—I was goin' to get the bairns immunised [late] by Dr Hamish and then it started oot aboot the whooping-cough needle givin' them brain damage and that was the end o't. And they're not helping the mothers of these babies any.(M16)

A fourth mother rejected immunisation for her daughter, since an older boy (only partly protected) had been feverish for a few days after his injection, developed measles despite immunisation, and appeared to be less healthy than his non-immunised sister. Nevertheless she allowed the boy to have his pre-school booster:

Well, they get it at school anyway—I just got it done. It's really the three needles they get when they are younger that I don't like—getting it so young.(M17)

She talked vaguely of a 'carry-on' concerning the whooping-cough injection, but admitted that this was not really her main objection.

It is perhaps discouraging that despite the efforts of health visitors imperfect immunisation records can still be found in this social group. However, it is clear that many of these mothers had thought about the matter in a reasoned way, but felt that sufficient information and opportunities for debate had not been made available. The controversies had certainly had an influence on their attitudes. Problems arise when information is presented by the mass media only, perhaps in a sensational way, and when the medical profession and health visitors do not have the time or the desire to discuss the question further. This is exacerbated by the division of responsibility between local authority clinic and GP. Better access to facilities would also improve the uptake in some cases. It is also clear, however, that a few mothers would never have their children immunised, since they consider prevention to be irrelevant for their 'healthy' offspring.

References

[1] Davie, R., Butler, N. and Goldstein, H. (1972), *From Birth to Seven: the Second Report of the National Child Development Study (1958 Cohort)*, London: Longman.

[2] Wedge, P. and Prosser, H. (1973), *Born to Fail?* London: Arrow Books and the National Children's Bureau.

[3] Butler, N. R. (1977), 'Community and family influences on 0 to fives: utilisation of pre-school day care and preventive health care', *Child Health and Education in the Seventies*, mimeo, University of Bristol and the National Birthday Trust Fund.

[4] *Scottish Health Statistics*, (1978), Edinburgh: HMSO.

11 Fertility Control

Most of the literature on this topic indicates that the poorest groups in society had, in the past, larger and less planned families than the rest of the population, for a variety of cultural and structural reasons.[1] This is obviously relevant to the possible perpetuation of deprivation. Since the average family size of our social class IV and V sample is 2.4 children, it is clear that for our group (as in Britain generally) the fertility differential between social classes appears to be less pronouned that it used to be, and that important changes have occurred since the childbearing years of their mothers. With our small sample, we cannot match the detailed exploration of family-building patterns of, for instance, Askham,[2] or Thompson and Illsley,[3] but a description of the women's point of view may be of interest.

The Grandmothers
The distribution of family sizes in each generation was shown in Table 3.1: these women had on average four children, and several bore six or more. In the 1950–53 data it appeared that this generation did tend to *want* slightly larger families; several women interviewed at the time of their first pregnancy planned to have at least four children. Nevertheless, many of the women who started off married life with the intention of limiting their family to one, two or three children, ended up with many more, often within a short space of time:

> It just happened. We wis actually just goin' to have one, an' we hid another eight.(G4)

Oral contraception was not in existence, other methods were considered unpleasant, bothersome, and often highly dependent on the husband's co-operation, and the clinics were felt to be embarrassing:

> In my days we didnae get nuthin'. You hid to go to the clinic for a cap and things like that. But there wis nae pills at that time. I went after I had three—got fitted for this cap. Sometimes I used it, sometimes no.(G3—five children)
> It wis embarrissin' goin' doon to the clinic. It's nae fit it is now,

they just walk in an' say 'Put me on the Pill.' But doon there
they'd poke about at you an' a'—well, you just didnae fancy gaun
there.(G23)

From the earlier data it is clear that contraception frequently
involved the husband 'being careful', i.e. coitus interruptus, and that
this was notable for its lack of success. Indeed, the interviewers
mentioned a considerable degree of 'fatalism' in relation to the contraceptive practices of this group of social class IV and V women.

Furthermore, in the grandmothers' youth not only was contraception less convenient, safe and freely available, but sterilisation
was much more difficult to obtain than at present, although
probably more common in the particular region of the study than in
other parts of the country. A psychiatric report was obtained on all
women who were referred for sterilisation. Despite their obviously
difficult circumstances in the past, only a quarter of the grandmothers on whom we have relevant information have been sterilised:

The social worker took down notes of what your wages were, what
you spent, if you had hire purchase.(G41)
Nowadays, if you carry your children wi' high blood pressure they
sterilise you. But in my day they didn't. (G3—severe high blood
pressure)

Several talked of their struggle to obtain sterilisation after seven or
eight pregnancies: 'But the sister on the ward says "Oh, you're too
healthy to be sterilised." ' (G4). G12, a mother of six children, whose
husband was violent, said she was told: 'You're quite a healthy
young person. Don't you want to practise birth control?'

However, a slight relaxation of attitude was noted over the years,
and several of our younger grandmothers, i.e. those in their forties,
appeared to have obtained sterilisation more easily. Nevertheless the
climate of opinion was very different from that of today and the
grounds of multiparity, debility, and emotional problems on which
the operation was performed had to be very clear:

I had four children in 3 years an' 8 months, an' I was headin' for a
nervous breakdown. Dr E. advised it. I had a hysterectomy before
I was 25. I was expecting a baby and I got it taken off.(G23)

It would be wrong to exaggerate the 'fatalism' and lack of control
over fertility in the grandmother generation, however. Some women
appeared to use the cap or sheath with a great deal of success and
limited their family to two or three children as they had planned.
G30 was fairly typical of several of the younger grandmothers,
though certainly not typical of the whole sample:

We took precautions. Put it this way, it was either do without a lot
of things and have a child sooner, or wait the gap and get what we
wanted first. So that's what we did—so that we could give the
family the benefit as well.(G30)

The Mothers

Despite the very high rate of illegitimate and prenuptial conception
among the young women—very few appeared to have used any form
of contraception before marriage—most of them had firm ideas
about the size of family they wanted or thought appropriate for
people like themselves. They had no intention of repeating the high
fertility patterns of their mothers' generation:

> I dinna want a big family, it's too expensive. Three's enough. I
> just put it in my mind then, whenever she was born (3rd child). I
> said nae mair kids for me.(M1)
> I had trouble with G. and I've got enough anyway. Three children
> is an odd number and I certainly wouldn't like four.(M38)
> When it was time to stop, it was time to stop. Three is
> enough.(M5)

Several of the women also gave the impression of being very much in
control of the timing of conception:

> I wasn't ready for children when I first got married. I wanted to
> save for everything for my house. I think you are more contented
> as a mother—you have more time for them.(M37)
> I was engaged at 16, married at 18, had M. at 20 and S. at 22. I'll
> only be 36 when M. is 16. We felt we would still be young when they
> were grown up.(M38)

However, it was quite common for the husband and wife to disagree
about how many children they should have, with perhaps the man
slightly more often wanting a larger family than the woman:

> But I said that after his job was finished I had to carry it for 9
> months and give birth to it!(M29)

Although many of the women succeeded in achieving the family size
and spacing they said they had initially desired or vaguely
imagined—by using contraception, being sterilised or experiencing
sub-fertility—for quite a few the reality was slightly different. Their
control over their fertility was rather less perfect than they wished,
due either to their own shortcomings or less frequently those of the
method of contraception chosen.

> Well, I wisnae planning on 3 kids—they was all really mistakes. I
> would sort of run out of the Pill—like it was my ain fault because I
> would probably wait until I'd finished my last packet.(M1)

W. [after an illegitimate child and prenuptial conception] was a mistake. I was working on night shift and sometimes forgot it [Pill].(M3)
I had B. before I was married, then I had M. That was to be the last. This one was a mistake. If I had my time over again, I wouldn't have family—22 with 3 kids. They say children make a marriage but I don't think so.(M9)

Several women who were adamant that they wanted no more children, or were 'terrified' of enduring another pregnancy, nevertheless spoke of very erratic contraceptive practices or of using no form of birth control at all. The concept of fatalism does, in these cases, seem to be relevant:[4]

If I fall, I fall. I'm just chancing it, but we can't really afford another.(M17)

M13, with three children and another due, said:

None of my family were planned. A speaker at our Mothers' Club went on about couples deciding if they can afford it, then planning a baby. If you are pregnant you just have to manage.(M13)

Another who had three children was adamant that her family was complete, but did not return to the clinic to have a coil inserted:

I've always meant to go but I've never got round to it. I couldn't be bothered.(M27)

Nevertheless it would be wrong to assert that all the couples in the sample with the largest families had an apathetic approach to birth control. Couples wanted more children for a variety of reasons; several said they stopped at two or three children *only* because of their financial situation:

Well, if there was lots of money, I'd think about another—it's the money really.(M64)

Commonly couples desired to have children of both sexes, e.g. one who had been sterilised after her third boy lamented:

I wept because he wasn't a girl. But I wasn't prepared to go on trying. I might have ended up with a football team!(M51)

M52 had her fourth child because they wanted a boy and her husband was extremely fond of children, as did M2: 'He wants a boy, and his happiness has to be considered too.' M53 felt that a fourth child would be a good idea, because she believed that the age-gap between the second and third children, due to frequent miscarriages, was too great. M14—pregnant again at 23, with four live children, and a history of miscarriage and termination—had absolutely no regrets about her situation:

> I want a big family. We were planning one soon anyway. I'm quite happy. If I wasn't, I'd just get sterilised.

Thus, despite some evidence that some of the women did not achieve the exact family composition and size they desired, there appeared to be no longer any need for them to have *many* more children than they wanted, since effective contraception was freely available.

It was true, however, that greater than average family size (i.e. more than two children) was associated with the categorisation of the families as 'more' or 'less' disadvantaged (see Table 11.1).

Table 11.1   Relationship of family size and index of 'disadvantage' of the family

	Families categorised as			
	'More disadvantaged'		'Less disadvantaged'	
1 or 2 children	11	(38%)	22	(76%)
3 or more children	18	(62%)	7	(24%)
(N = 100%)	(29)		(29)	

The women who have been quoted as expressing fatalistic attitudes were likely to be in the 'more disadvantaged' group. It must be noted, however, that this relationship is more problematic, in this complex area of fertility behaviour, than it is in some of the other areas of health behaviour which have been examined. Even among the 'more disadvantaged', large families were in some cases a deliberate choice rather than any indication of fatalistic attitudes and lack of control. There does remain a group, however, who appeared to be less able to remain in control of their fertility.

Methods of Contraception

Almost every woman in our sample had at some time used oral contraception, including at least one insulin diabetic. One wife of a Catholic never used the Pill, while another Catholic husband wholeheartedly approved of the practice. For most it was the only form of contraception offered or considered, and was believed to be the safest:

> They [hospital] wanted me to take the Pill.(M28)
> They send you awa' [from hospital] with the Pill in your hand.(M55)
> I don't think any young woman uses any form of contraception apart from the Pill.(M8)

Most preferred to obtain oral contraceptives on prescription from their GP rather than attend the local family planning clinics; they reported that this involved less embarrassment and delay:

> I would sort of run out of the Pill and then if you phone up the Family Planning—'Oh, I'm sorry.' You could nae get an appointment till next week—so I just ging to my doctor now.(M1)

Very few of the women considered, or used, the sheath, coil or cap, and several expressed extreme distaste at the thought of having any device inserted, or discussed 'scares' about side effects. Only three women mentioned using the sheath, although there may have been considerable under-reporting. Women, through necessity or preference, generally took action on their own or faced the consequences: one grandmother made this rather bitter comment on the failings of her son-in-law:

> And her husband wouldnae use any other type of contraceptive. So, I mean, she just became pregnant, it was the only alternative.(G29)

and another woman who was determined to retain control of her fertility said:

> He doesnae believe in the Pill either—you'd have ten kids or something [i.e. if left to the husband].(M1)

Despite the high rate of oral contraceptive use among our sample, almost all of the women were either apprehensive about its long-term consequences, were bothered by immediate side effects, or in some way believed that the Pill was 'unnatural'. Many reported that they had experienced weight gain or loss, tiredness, severe headaches, nausea, bad temper, more frequent menstruation, pain in legs or stomach, high blood pressure, constipation, fluid retention, the onset of clinical diabetes (reported medical diagnosis). We can only take reports of these symptoms at face value, although in some cases these claims may have been a means of obtaining speedy sterilisation, an 'excuse' to stop using something of which they disapproved, or a 'legitimate' reason for having more children than professionals such as health visitors thought acceptable, or the families could afford:

> It made me really irritable. R. [husband] and I were not getting on. He just had to come home and say something to me and I'd blow up. Well, it's not worth breaking a marriage over a little pill.(M13)

Most of the women were offered several brands to alleviate the numerous side effects suffered but several eventually became discouraged.

It is clear that publicity and 'scares' surrounding the long-term effects of prolonged use of oral contraception had reached this section of the population and created some distress:

> I read in the Sunday papers about women having blood clots and strokes and going blind. In America they have warnings about this on the packets. In Britain they only tell you about the small side effects like headaches and depression. I was so worried. I wasn't sure whether I should start the next packet.(M28)

However, fear of problems arising in the future appeared to be a less important factor in influencing women's decisions to stop taking the Pill than the more immediate side effects. Several women (or their husbands) felt that oral contraception was 'unnatural' and therefore bound to produce unintended consequences:

> It interferes with nature when it shouldn't.(M14)
> I'm not a Roman Catholic or anything, but maybe I'm just old-fashioned, but I dinna like the idea of the Pill. It must do something to your body. I've heard of women whose periods didnae come back for years when they came off it—that proves it—or bleeding all the time—shows it must do something to you—it's unnatural.(M61)

If there was such a degree of uncertainty about oral contraception and distaste for other methods of birth control, how did these women succeed in limiting their family size? For many, sterilisation was the most obvious solution to fear of being on the Pill for the rest of their fertile lives.

Sterilisation

The numbers of sterilisations performed in the City have grown rapidly in recent years, and occur at younger ages and at lower parity.[5] This operation was offered to, or requested by, the women in our sample in what appeared to be a routine way. Twenty-two of the mothers were sterilised, usually post-partum, and three of the husbands had had a vasectomy, i.e. there were 25 families (43 per cent) where one partner had been sterilised. A further nine women wished to be sterilised—they asked their general practitioner and the request had gone no further, or they were on the hospital waiting list—and seven had been offered sterilisation and had refused the procedure.

The average age at sterilisation among the sample was 24, after bearing an average of 2.5 children. Very early operations were usually performed on medical grounds, e.g. one woman was only 17 when her husband (who suffered from a hereditary condition) had a vasectomy, and a woman of 20 had 'kidney trouble'. However, it was not uncommon for the women to be sterilised, or offered the operation, at 21 or 22 after having three children, or at 23 years of age after two:

> When I was in ha'in' my second een—'Well, are you going to be sterilised?'—Shock!(M12)

Two female sterilisations and two vasectomies were carried out when there was only one child of the couple.

Sterilisation had become so much part of life in the City that for many women it was an automatic request after having two or three children. Operations for medical reasons were still performed, and were represented amongst our sample as we have seen, but they were in the minority. More typical were the following comments:

> And then when I fell wi' L., I asked to get sterilised. That was the finish.(M4)
> My husband and I discussed it and decided it was the best plan.(M7)
> I didn't want to go back on the Pill, so I asked to be sterilised.(M8)

Few of these women appeared to regret their decision, and indicated that they were given plenty of time to change their minds. (Several of the others in the sample did in fact back out at the last minute.) However, one unfortunate case of a divorced mother is worth quoting, although she may have been reconstructing what actually happened:

> I wish I hadna now, but it canna be helped. There was no problems getting done, but the city's known for that. I was lying there, and I thought 'No, I'm no sure about this.' And nobody seems to talk to you. I think they should. I never got somebody who came to me and said 'Do you want this?' If they had I would have said 'No'. As it turns out it was a mistake—I dinna think I can marry anyone else now, with not being able to have more family, it wouldn't be fair.(M70)

Three of the four women with four children had turned down the operation (for many of the reasons connected with family size discussed earlier), despite some pressure from health visitors and general practitioners:

> I might think about it if I was older. But if I got sterilised, every time I saw a baby I'd just cry. (M52, aged 24 with 4 children)
> I would never get that done even if I had 10 children. After the third one [at 19] they advised me to get sterilised, and I was thinking about it because I had such a bad time, but my husband said I would regret it, to wait a few months. It was a good job I

didn't get it done, because in a few weeks I'd forgotten about it. I thought I was too young.(M14)

Undoubtedly among the most vociferous of our sample were the women who said they had requested sterilisation and claimed they had been turned down. We have, of course, no independent information about what actually happened in these cases, but it appeared that these women were in very similar circumstances to those for whom sterilisation had been almost part of a routine process. However, this may reflect a more recent decision by consultants to delay sterilisation if in any doubt, and to an increase, for various reasons, in the length of waiting lists. In addition, some of the women may have made their request to inappropriate hospital staff who were unable to deal with it. Among examples of these women was one who presented herself as financially insecure, who said that she was refused sterilisation after two children at the age of 20, then again at 23 after her third child (fourth pregnancy):

> They said to me 'You're a healthy woman. You could have another ten children.' And I said 'Are you going to look after them and clothe them?' Even my husband agrees that three children is too many. But I just said that if I fall pregnant again, I'm going to have it taken from me. Even suppose I'm in for ten abortions.(M13)

She did become pregnant again, but attended for antenatal care so late that abortion was out of the question; she had changed her mind in any case. Another woman, aged 22 with two children, presented a similar case, but her request got no further than her GP. Like most of the women in this situation, she had formulated her own ideas about consultants' decision-rules for sterilisation. When pregnant once more she commented:

> They'll do me now because this is my third one. They won't do you at 22 with two.(M17)

Despite support from her health visitor, the woman's hopes were not fulfilled. A third woman became pregnant while on the Pill, after her GP refused to refer her for sterilisation at 24 after two difficult and premature deliveries, and her dismay was increased when her husband, requesting a vasectomy in order to spare her further trauma, was told by his GP that it would be simpler for his wife to undergo sterilisation after the third child was born:

> He didn't even discuss it. I don't know why they are going to invent these things if doctors aren't going to allow them. I just felt that everything was put on my shoulders, left to the wife again.(M38)

Nevertheless, despite these few cases where the women felt that control of their fertility was being taken out of their hands, it is clear that our sample had quite definite ideas about the size of family with which they could cope, and had, to a greater extent, been provided with the means—through contraception and sterilisation—of carrying out their plans.

References

[1] e.g. Rainwater, L. (1960), *And the Poor Get Children*, Chicago, Ill.: Quadrangle Books.

[2] Askham, J. (1975), *Fertility and Deprivation*, Cambridge: Cambridge University Press.

[3] e.g. Thompson, B. and Illsley, R. (1969), 'Family growth in Aberdeen', *J. Biosoc. Sci.*, **1**, 28–38

[4] See Chamberlain, A. (1976), 'Planning versus fatalism', *J. Biosoc Sci.*, **8**, 1–16.

[5] Thompson, B. and Aitken-Swan, J. (1973), 'Pregnancy outcome and fertility control in Aberdeen', *Brit. J. Prev. Soc. Med.*, **27**, 137.
Nottage, B. J., Hall, M. H. and Thompson, B. (1977), 'Social and medical trends in female sterilisation in Aberdeen 1951–72', *J. Biosoc. Sci.*, **9**, 487–500.

12 Infant Feeding and Child Nutrition

This section considers the views and practices of both generations concerning nutrition, and its relationship to the health of the children. Both grandmothers and mothers were asked whether they had breast- or bottle-fed their children and what their reasons had been. The grandmothers' accounts could be compared with the data from the 1950–53 study, and the mothers' with maternity and health visitor records. The weaning of infants was directly relevant only in the families with young babies at the time of our survey, and we did not obtain systematic information about this stage from the other mothers or the grandmothers. The topic was sometimes raised spontaneously, however, and since it was a particular point of conflict which some mothers talked about or which was recorded in the health visitor records, it seems worthy of special discussion.

Infant Feeding
Fashions in breast- or bottle-feeding have, of course, swung to and fro during the period of time represented by our two generations. Despite the evidence for the benefits of breast-feeding and the official policy regarding its promotion, actual practices of encouragement carried out by doctors or health visitors at different times or in different places may also vary. For a long time it has been one cause for concern, however, that women in the lower social classes have been thought to breast-feed less. This was found to be true in the National Survey of Health and Development, at a period before our grandmother generation were having their children;[1] equally it was true in the National Child Development Survey at a time nearer the childbearing of our mother generation. In the NCDS, 79 per cent of mothers in social class I breast-fed initially, compared with 64 per cent of social class V, and these proportions had fallen at one month after birth to 59 per cent and 36 per cent.[2]

The proportions of breast-feeding mothers in both our generations are shown in Table 12.1, and it can be noted that in the present generation, in this area and this social group, breast-feeding was

Table 12.1   Proportion of women breast-feeding, per cent

| | Grandmothers[a] | Mothers | |
	First child	First child	Latest child where more than one
Full breast-feeding	28	(1)	4
Breast-feeding for at least 14 days	28	(1)	4
Breast-feeding for less than 14 days	31	(1)	9
Bottle-feeding	14	95	83
(N = 100%)	(29)	(58)	(54)

Note: [a] Only those on whom 1950–53 data exists

found to be even less common than in the social class V mothers of the NCDS.

The grandmothers

At the time when our grandmothers had their first children, an attempt to breast-feed was mandatory in the hospital concerned, unless there were contrary medical factors or the mother was extremely determined to bottle-feed. Some of our grandmothers remembered this policy clearly:

> I didn't want to breast-feed. This lady in the bed next to me, she was bottle. I says why is *she* getting a bottle for her baby? So the nurse, she stood up and she said, Listen, ladies, this is a young mother of 24 who wants to bottle-feed her first baby! Well, I felt very—and she says, that's *her* eighth child. Oh, I really felt terrible. So I said, all right, then I'll do it. And I did.(G33)

As Table 12.1 shows, however, many of our grandmothers gave up soon after returning home. It may also be noted that breast-feeding for children subsequent to the first was reported to us as less common. In their accounts to us, the majority offered medical reasons or physiological failures—illnesses of the baby, breast abscesses, 'the milk ran out', 'they weren't getting the good of it', 'I just had dishwater.' A few explained that they were working, or their own mother was caring for the child from the beginning. Only one said that she was determined to bottle-feed from the first, and did.

Our grandmothers are, of course, a small group from the much larger 1950–53 survey. We may relate what individuals told us, some 30 years later, to the information recorded then. We may also relate our group to the general findings of the original study, to see whether our grandmothers are atypical in any way.

In general, it appears that our grandmothers were giving us very accurate accounts. We can make the direct comparison in 21 cases (30 families from the 1950–53 survey, less two sisters, one case where there was no information on breast-feeding in the original survey, two cases where the mother-in-law was interviewed in the place of an absent mother, and four grandmothers who refused interviews). In only two of these is there any discrepancy at all about the facts. In one case a grandmother told us that she was never able to breast-feed: 'I had plenty of milk, but nothing nourishing, it was just fluid' (G29) although the earlier records suggest that she breast-fed her daughter for 10 weeks. The second woman gave the reason for ceasing after a very short period that she was working, though the records give the cause as mastitis (G31). For the rest, the stories agree in every detail with the earlier records, which would appear to be remarkable evidence of truthfulness and long memory.

Our group as a whole may be compared with 186 married women having their first child booked for confinement in the maternity hospital in 1953, whose antenatal attitudes to infant feeding and subsequent practices were studied.[3] Of the 159 women who had a live child and were available 3 months after their confinement, 22 were unable to breast-feed. Of the rest, over one-quarter gave up before the baby was a month old, and just over two-fifths were still feeding at 13 weeks. 'Unskilled manual and fish-trade workers' were less likely than other occupational groups to continue to feed after 13 weeks—28 per cent, compared with 52 per cent of 'professional, technical and clerical workers'. Thus, it seems that our group of social class IV/V women was not atypical.

The attitudes to breast-feeding of the majority of the grandmothers now were equivocal (see Table 12.2). Yes, it was said to be healthier for the baby, and it might be less trouble and expense. But 'if you're working it might be a pest I would think' (G32), 'you haven't such a good social life' (G41) and, in any case, 'nowadays young girls just dinna want to feed babies, it's dying out' (G29); 'The young ones won't do it now. They want to get out in the evenings, it ties them in.' (G68) In general, they gave the impression that they would not want to judge, for young mothers now, because they should make their own decisions:

> They'll tell you you should breast-feed your baby. Now, I dinna think they should be in a position to tell you fit to dee, because efter a' it's your baby.(G13)

A minority of grandmothers, not all of whom had breast-fed their own daughters for more than a brief period, were eloquent about the

Table 12.2   Grandmothers' current attitudes to breast-feeding

	Per cent
Enthusiastic—would always recommend it	19
Neutral—advantages and disadvantages, no views expressed	72
Only negative views expressed	9
(N = 100%)	(47)

advantages of breast-feeding. Usually they appealed to emotional advantages first, and practical or health advantages only secondarily:

> It's a natural thing, I mean if you watch the television, if you watch a baby being breast-fed by its mother, you can see the contentment, actual contentment on that bairn's face . . . I think it's bonny to see a baby being fed that way.(G40)
> . . . and the majority of them I've noticed seem to be closer, you know, to their mothers. And then it's a natural food, you haven't the problem of is the milk too hot or too cold.(G37)

The small minority who were definitely against breast-feeding may be illustrated by the grandmother who said yes, she had breast-fed her children, but that was

> . . . old-fashioned now. I thought that that was the natural thing to do. I think they're better bottle-fed. You know what they're getting with a bottle or maybe your milk wouldnae be up to standard, and you wouldn't know, would you? I mean it's the baby that suffers.(G34)

The mothers

As Table 12.1 showed, a much smaller proportion of the mothers had ever attempted to breast-feed any of their children—only 9 of the 58 mothers, for 14 of the 139 children. This information given to us by the mothers agreed completely with that in the records. In contrast to the grandmothers, who had often fed only their first, the mothers were more likely to have attempted some breast-feeding for a second or third child rather than the first.

There is little point in a close analysis of the reasons which the women gave for not breast-feeding, for most of them were obviously offering us selections from what they saw as the available explanations: the baby was in the Special Nursery, they were not able to, bottle-feeding was more practical or convenient, they were intending to go back to work, the demands of other small children made it too difficult, and so on.

Table 12.3   Mothers' current attitudes to breast-feeding

	Per cent
Those who did, for at least one child (16 per cent):	
Favourable	9
Regrets breast-feeding, or did not succeed for more than a few days	7
Those who did not (84 per cent)	
Says she wanted to, or tried, but was unable to	12
Now says that she wishes she had	5
Has no regrets about bottle-feeding	67
(N = 100%)	(58)

As Table 12.3 shows, few of them regretted bottle-feeding or giving up breast-feeding after only a few days; the great majority were matter-of-fact about their decision and said simply (or in addition to other explanations) that they 'never had any inclination', 'never thought of it', 'didn't like the idea of it', or 'just never fancied it'.

Despite the fact that the promotion of breast-feeding is still the formal policy of the maternity hospitals, and that health visitors reported that they always discussed it pre-natally and encouraged it, the young mothers gave the general impression that their decisions were accepted without comment. They said, 'They don't pressure you to breast-feed in hospital now' or, commonly, 'They just ask you', 'They let you please yourself.' The only woman who remembered any pressure at all similar to that reported by the grand-mothers said that, when she had her first child:

> I remember there was a sister there, and she raved at me—there's milk there, she says, and I says I'm nae worried if there's milk there, I just don't want to. This last time they just asked, breast or bottle? and I said, I bottle-feed, and they didn't say anything.(M68)

One health visitor said in interview that though she always recommended breast-feeding, she would never press a mother who was clearly against it, 'because it's never successful then' and indeed it seemed that pressure might be counter-productive, for a few mothers said that they 'went off the idea' because of 'everyone going on about what a good idea it was'. On the other hand, two of the women who wanted to breast-feed complained that they did not get enough support and help, possibly because the hospital staff were too busy: the account of one was:

There I was, they put you behind the curtain and no one comes near, I was greeting [crying] away. I had plenty of milk but I didn't know how to make him take it, plenty of milk but nae help.(M70)

A majority of the mothers, however, were very definitely against breast-feeding. Two themes in their discussion of it are perhaps of interest. The first relates to the way in which the women perceive their own bodies, and the revulsion that some of them expressed at the idea of a baby feeding from them. They almost gave the impression that, to them, bottle-feeding was cleaner (several mentioned the staining of clothes with breast milk) and more *natural*:

I didn't really want to, anyway, but if I had I would have been put right off by the girl I shared a room with. She was feeding and she was all swollen and enormous, it was horrible. She kept on having to squeeze the milk into a bowl—I couldn't watch, it made me sick.(M67)

As one mother said:

You didn't associate your breasts with feeding. They were sort of part of your figure.(M32)

and several discussed breast-feeding primarily in relation to the effect that it had, or might have, upon their figure. Two of those who had fed a child but were not enthusiastic about the experience said: 'I wouldn't do it again. I ended up with no bust' (M18) and, on the other hand, 'I thought it would help to reduce my bust and trim my figure, but it didn't work.' (M17)

The second theme, perhaps related to the first, is the acute embarrassment that many of the mothers expressed about breast-feeding. A high proportion—nearly 20 per cent—gave it as one of their principle objections:

I wouldn't like to do it in front of my own husband, never mind anyone else. I wouldn't do it in front of my sister-in-law, and she comes in every day. And if a crowd of people came in, you couldn't just sit and breast-feed, so you'd have to go into another room and everyone would know why.(M13)

A few grandmothers had felt the same, but they tended to suggest that 'things were different now'—despite the fact that, in our interviews, it was the young mothers who more frequently mentioned it. As one grandmother explained:

I said til her, the best thing she could dee would be to breast-feed, and she says it would curb her activities, ken, she has a' this squash and badminton and things like this. I said, Och, it didnae need to curb you, you could still lead a normal life, even though you are breast-feeding. I says, there's naebody bothers now whether you're breast-feeding now, onywey, div they? People nowadays are mair open-minded aboot things, aren't they? Although I used to—I've seen me sitting in the dark, ken, as long as it wis in the corner, naebody saw you. That's my attitude, and I've been trying to pass it on to them.(G70)

Another grandmother made a comment with an interesting use of the word 'disgrace': 'Oh yes, I'd recommend it. There's no *disgrace* in it, none whatsoever.' (G30) On the whole, however, the grandmothers gave the impression that—since health professionals were not so insistent nowadays—the question of breast-feeding was not one they were prepared to be dogmatic about. One or two of them, and one health visitor, said that they thought it was 'coming back' when compared with the more recent past. The evidence that more of our mothers had breast-fed a subsequent child than at first (Table 12.1) may support this.

The Weaning of Infants

In discussing their infant feeding experience, three mothers made interesting comments to the effect that (though breast-feeding was said to be preferable) it had not mattered that they bottle-fed their babies, because 'they weren't on the bottle long, anyway' or 'they were off the bottle very early so it was OK'.

If grandmothers were unlikely, in the accounts given to us, to influence their daughters with regard to breast- or bottle-feeding, the question of early supplementation and weaning may have been different. When the grandmothers were having their children the early feeding of cereal or solids was not so firmly discouraged, and they certainly described early supplementation: one alleged that her doctor told her, when the baby was three weeks old, to put her onto 'Co-op' milk with 'Bengers and Virol' added to it. A few grandmothers did describe how they advised their daughters:

E. was ten weeks old and sometimes she'd cry before her feed's due and I'll say, why don't you give her a rich tea biscuit rolled with some hot milk and a half teaspoon of sugar? She's ten week, I feel maybe now she wants something more solid.(G22)

The mothers, however, usually insisted that they were making their own decisions and using their own common sense:

You were told this and you were told that—but you know when your bairn's hungry and wants some more.(M37)
I just did what I wanted.(M54)

These decisions were, however, one of the greatest sources of con-flict with health visitors and clinic doctors. The health visitors' notes were full of criticism about overfeeding, adding 'extra' milk powder, giving full-cream milk or cow's milk too early, feeding cereal and other solids at a few weeks, or, as one health visitor (some years ago) had despairingly noted in the child's records:

insisting on feeding cow's milk, pudding, raw eggs and other rubbish to the child [at 4 months]. Mother not amenable to advice.

The majority of mothers certainly did believe in early mixed feeding. We observed infants of two months being spoon-fed, cereal being given at 6 weeks, or in the case of another 6-week-old baby a mother reported:

She eats anything. I just put what we're having in the liquidiser. She has all sorts of things—I like to let her taste lots of different things.(M68)

Unfortunately, however, the conflict that arose was the cause of several mothers having given up going to clinics, or refusing to pay attention to their health visitor's general advice. They felt that they 'knew' what their baby wanted, and that if more food or more solids 'cured' a baby that had been in the habit of crying all night, then it was clear proof that this had been the right course of action. In any case, they might well be desperate—with husbands and perhaps other small children to consider—and ready to try any remedy for a seemingly discontented infant. Early supplementation, or early weaning, manifestly 'worked': though the mothers might have been told of the possible disadvantages, they were not immediate and obvious. There was no evidence that they had retained much of what they had been told—if indeed they had—about the medical reasons for current policy.

A typical account given by a mother was:

When I told the health visitor [about giving cereal at 3 weeks] she went off her head. She said she was too young. I said, I'm going to feed her the way I want to feed her!(M30)

In other cases, the mother was concealing her practices from the health visitor:

When I came home I put him onto full cream and half a rusk. Miss X didn't like that! So I stopped telling her. She'd say, now you're only giving him his bottle, aren't you? And I'd say, yes, yes! But at six weeks I'd give C. the yolk of an egg—he just loved it.(M5)

This conflict was obviously harmful to the relationship between mother and health visitor, and might turn the mother against professional advisers in general: several women described how they refused to use clinics because 'I always get into trouble for giving them the wrong things' (M53) or refused to go back after a particular occasion when, as it seemed to them, no solution had been offered for their problems:

> ... she was only weeks old, and she was always crying ... they told me to give her more milk, but I told them that wouldn't help, because she didn't even empty the bottle that I gave her, she was wanting something more filling.(M18)
> The milk he was put on didn't agree with him, he was always hungry. They wouldn't believe he was wanting feeding five times in an evening ... I haven't gone back.(M54)

Child Nutrition

Finally, we analyse the more general ideas about the nutrition of children presented by both generations. They were all asked 'What do you think keeps children healthy?' or 'Have you any special recipes for keeping children healthy?' Many of them would include some comments about food in their answer, indicating that food was, to them, a salient component of health care. If they did not mention food, we would follow up with a supplementary question, 'What about food?', and if they still did not go into any detail we would press them, 'What sort of foods do you think are good for children?'

We thus have *accounts*, from both generations, of their knowledge and ideas about nutrition. We have little evidence, for either grandmothers or mothers, of the relationship these bear to actual practices, past or present. It must be made clear that we have no complete or reliable record of the diets of the survey children. To the mothers' accounts we can, however, add the comments of health visitors and the results of our own observation, in order to make some judgement about any obvious discrepancies between accounts and practices.

The grandmothers

About one third of the grandmothers did not spontaneously mention food as important for children's health, or said that they had no particular views on the subject: 'Mine just ate a'thing that wis goin'!' (G23) The majority, however, were enthusiastic on the subject, often quoting the remembered wisdom of *their* parents:

> My father aye said if you've got a fire and a diet o' meat you winna hae a'thing, you'll aye be a'right.(G13)

My mother was always good, you know, and she used to always say, put good food into them when they're young, because you canna put it into them when they're old.(G22)

Table 12.4 shows which foods were mentioned as 'good' by each generation. In general, the main emphasis of the grandmothers was upon plain, solid food:

A cooked solid meal.(G2)
Soup and sweet, meat and potatoes, regular meals, not too much in between.(G10)
... your usual meals like most families, I mean, your soups, your potato, your meat and your pudding.(G38)

'Proper' meals of this sort were opposed to snacks and sweets, which were perceived as all too common among the younger generation:

They're feeding bairns all this rubbish nowadays.(G14)
Good nourishing food, instead of all that snackery they get, sweets and things.(G11)
They give him anything he wants and if he doesn't want his dinner they don't push him. Which I quite agree with, you canna push a child to eat. But then, I wouldn't give him sweets—he's filled up with sweets.(G22)

Table 12.4   Foods which are 'good' for children

	Grandmother	Mother
	Per cent giving this answer	
Milk	9	47
Eggs	11	33
Cheese	7	14
Meat	30	19
Potatoes	24	—
Other vegetables	22	21
Fruit	13	31
Fish	15	12
Soup	28	9
Cereals, oatcakes	7	5
Porridge	17	3
Steamed/milk puddings	11	—
(N = 100%)	(47)	(58)

(Other examples mentioned by one or two women)

Table 12.4 shows that the grandmothers believed strongly in meat, which they usually specified as beef, 'mince and tatties', or 'good' meat. They were also enthusiastic about vegetables: 'I'm aye telling her, give them cabbage! Give them carrot an' neap!', but they reserved the greatest eloquence for a combination of the two in home-made soups: 'Plenty soup, made wi' good stock. Plenty o' vitamins in that.' (G22)

They praised 'good broth' on grounds of economy as well as nutrition:

> Soup was the cheapest thing to make at that time.(G41)
> My mither could never hae bought four tins, five tins o' soup to pit in a pot!(G19)

but the notable theme running through their comments was of some concept of 'goodness'. There were foods that were full of good-ness—an inherent quality related to nutritive value but rather more than that. Goodness was connected with naturalness, purity, home preparation rather than commercial processing, lack of adulteration and 'chemicals'. Meat bones and fresh vegetables, boiled for a long time, contained the essence of this goodness and moral virtue attached to the housewife who obtained it for her family. Tinned foods, and especially tinned soup, could not contain it:

> There's nae nourishment in that. You're better with your own. A bone—you're getting goodness off a bone, the marrow out o' a bone.(G3)
> None of this tinned meat and artificial foods. And nothing out of a fridge! (Great-grandmother in family 9)
> You got baked rice. It was made wi' eggs and there wis currants in it, and this was a luxury, mind. Nowadays they get a tin and there's nae eggs in it and the goodness is out o' it. The things nowadays—the richt good is out o' them—the body-building material. Tinned soup—I would never hae it in the house. We wis brought up to get a'thing oot o' the ground and intae a pot.(G19)

Twelve of the respondents, or 26 per cent, specifically condemned tinned foods. Sometimes they appealed to their husband's taste:

> My husband doesn't like tins at a', he thinks there's a flavour, there's some funny flavouring in these things.(G63)

and sometimes they acknowledged that working mothers might not have time to cook:

> A lot of things are tinned, I suppose it's for convenience now, people working, but I still prefer the home-made soup, made with fresh vegetables. I think it's got a different taste.(G67)

but on the whole the inherent goodness of home-made foods required no defence. Frozen foods appeared not to have entered the grandmother's repertoire: it must be noted that only one grandmother, and only a few mothers, owned a deep-freeze cabinet or fridge-freezer.

More scientific notions about nutrition, or information which might have been obtained from the media or from contact with professional advisers, were rarely proffered. 'Roughage' was mentioned approvingly by one woman, and 'protein' by three (one of whom had some further education). 'Vitamins'—undifferentiated—were mentioned by six, often in connection with vegetables or fruit: 'Vitamins ... an apple a day to give them rosy cheeks.' (G6)

The mothers

We do not know what relationships these accounts given by the grandmothers bear to the *actual* diet of their children, in the circumstances of considerable poverty which many of them experienced in the 1950s. From the records and the mothers' accounts of their own health, it seems likely that many of them did in fact suffer from very poor nutrition. A quotation from one mother may illustrate this, and also demonstrate the very limited knowledge about nutrition which we found to be perhaps even more typical of the younger generation than the older:

> I took rickets as a child—nobody else in the family took rickets, I don't know why I took it, nobody seemed to have any idea. I could have been playing with someone who had it and passed it on.(M25)

Similarly, as noted earlier, we have little evidence about the actual diets of the survey children. On the whole, however, our observation suggested that the mothers were giving us an accurate picture of what their children ate, even where they knew diets were imperfect: they would either justify such diets ('I don't believe in fussing about food', 'After all, they're healthy') or explain the practical or economic problems which prevented a perfect diet.

Fewer mothers than grandmothers placed a high value upon nutrition as part of health care: less than half mentioned diet spontaneously when asked what keeps children healthy. The majority of the rest included food when pressed for an answer, though a few said specifically that 'what you ate made no difference'.

There was also less variety among the mothers, as shown in Table 12.4. With remarkable unanimity they recited milk, eggs, fruit, vegetables, meat as the foods which comprised a good diet. Milk was easily the most approved food for children, and it appeared to be true that most families consumed an adequate amount. Indeed, milk appeared to have a high symbolic value: a good mother was one who gave her children milk, no child could be ill-nourished who drank milk, milk was the universal food, the sign of plenty and well-being. To be without milk for the children was to demonstrate the worst fecklessness or destitution. One mother, talking about the advantages of close communities, expressed this well:

> If you have a family to help you, your baby need never starve. They would never refuse you milk. I know my family wouldn't. If I went to my mother and she had only half a pint of milk, she'd give it to me for the bairn and I'd get a cup of tea. Even if you don't have a family there is always a chum or a neighbour you could go to for milk for your bairn.(M13)

On the other hand, bread appeared to be completely demoted from its 'staff of life' image, and there was little reference to other cereal products—with very few mentions of porridge, compared to the older generation. Bread seemed almost to be a degrading food. One mother was ashamed because her child liked to eat bread ' . . . with nothing on it. I'm affronted in case anyone sees her. She doesn't even fold it over.' (M6). Another demonstrated how 'unfussy' her children were by saying 'It doesn't *have* to be biscuits. They'll eat a slice of bread and butter.' (M13)

If bread—and perhaps porridge—represented poverty and the 'bad old days', the representatives of prosperity were fruit and meat. Mothers said with pride 'sometimes they get fruit' or 'they get fruit every day' as evidence of a good diet, though there were some comments about fruit being too expensive to give as much as the mothers would have liked: 'They both eat fruit, but it's too dear to give them.' (M55) Meat, too, was a status symbol, though it must be noted that only about a quarter of the mothers mentioned it at all. A distinction was made between what is called, in Scotland, 'butchers meat' and tinned or prepared meats. Only a few of those mothers who said that meat was good specifically mentioned the beef, or mince, that contained the essence of 'goodness' for their own mothers. Stewed or roast meat was mentioned by only three mothers. For the rest, it was taken for granted that 'butcher's meat' was too expensive, or perhaps too difficult to prepare, and the actual meat products eaten were pies, hamburgers, sausages and tinned meats. Six families said specifically that the children ate no meat. In a fishing area, fish was perhaps surprisingly infrequently mentioned.

Vegetables, as Table 12.4 showed, were commonly mentioned as 'good'. On the other hand, they were also the item most frequently mentioned as something the children disliked and never ate. A list of all those foods said to be disliked is perhaps not important, as it is as varied and idiosyncratic as one might expect for young children. The only unanimity concerned fresh vegetables (excluding potatoes), which were never used in over a quarter of the families. In several cases it was alleged to be the father's taste which prevailed: he would not eat vegetables so the children copied him or the mother thought them not worth preparing. Potatoes were never specifically mentioned as a good food, though a great deal of chips and crisps were eaten. Salad vegetables were only once mentioned. The emphasis on fruit, and the neglect of vegetables (in an area where vegetables are easily grown or obtained and fruit expensive), represents a marked change since the generation before. Of course, few of these families had gardens of their own, and it is possible that vegetables, like bread (though acknowledged to be 'good for you'), had come to represent the bad old days of poverty.

Another change, perhaps for similar reasons, was the comparative neglect of that 'home-made soup' so universally lauded by the grand-mothers. Only seven families mentioned it, in two cases as a habit learned from the grandmothers, and in two others always actually made by her rather than by the young mother.

Only a minority of the mothers appeared to do very much cooking, and baking was superceded by the ubiquitous bakers' vans. They talked of 'made meals'—that is, cooked meals with potatoes, as opposed to ready-made or convenience foods—as something slightly unusual. Either they were proud of the fact that they were specially good housewives who made meals for their families—'My mother always made meals and so do I' (M37)—or they offered excuses—'I used to have made meals, but the children wouldn't eat them so I stopped.' (M21) Some mothers who prided themselves on being good cooks presented themselves as consciously being part of an older tradition:

> They like a'things home-made. My husband's like that, too, no' one for tins . . . quick meals. I cook meat, and F. gets the gravy. Maybe it doesn't make any difference to their health, mind you. I only do it probably because my granny aye did. And my husband's mother, she's a great cook, she wouldn't buy pies and that. I have to keep up! (M65)

Of course, many of the children had meals at their grandmother's, or lunches at school. With many mothers working, especially on evening jobs, or husbands away or working on shifts, the concept of a regular 'family meal' was not always appropriate. In several

families with an unemployed husband or one working different
hours to his wife, it was in fact the father who 'got the children's
tea'. There were some indications that 'made meals' were required
by men, but were not normal for women and children; as one single-
handed mother explained:

> It's difficult, when it's just you and the kids. You haven't got to
> make meat and that, so you don't—you get like them, eating
> rubbish all the time. My mum's always on about soups and that,
> but they don't like soup.(M70)

Most of the families agreed that they ate, and were observed to eat,
large quantities of tinned beans, tinned spaghetti, pies, ice-cream,
soft drinks, cakes, biscuits and baker's products generally, though
they did not defend these as part of a good diet. They were likely to
quote fatty foods and sweet foods, 'too much sugar', or 'cream
buns' as things which were bad for children. Like most parents of
most children, they had considerable problems in controlling the
intake of sweets and snacks. Even in the most extreme cases, where
the children were admitted (and observed) to spend the whole time
nibbling, the mothers usually acknowledged that this was 'bad', but
professed themselves unable to prevent it. Peer pressure when the
children went to school was responsible, or the grandparents or
father 'spoiled' the child. One mother explained this: 'He gives them
sweets because he never got, and he doesn't want them to do without.' (M27) The mothers had also to contend with a special hazard:
the travelling vans which toured the housing estates, offering regular
temptation to the child—and, indeed, the mother. 'She wants something from every van that comes around' was a common complaint,
and 'Our ice-cream van comes round three times of an evening.' For
whatever reason, our mothers found it very difficult to restrict sweet-
eating, though a minority did profess to try. Daily sums of 30–35
pence per child for snacks were not uncommon, with the consequences for dental decay which are described in Chapter 9.

About half the young infants were being given vitamin or orange-
juice supplements, but these were usually soon dropped as a mixed

Although, as has been noted, a proportion of the mothers had
very positive ideas about food and a keen sense of the value of good
nutrition, their theoretical knowledge appeared limited. While it
must be remembered that no specific questions were *asked* of them,
the information that they volunteered in explaining their food
preferences was rather meagre. No one mentioned the word
'protein'. 'Roughage' was mentioned approvingly by only one
mother. The only topic frequently introduced was 'vitamins'.

About half the young infants were being given vitamin or orange-
juice supplements, but these were usually soon dropped as a mixed

diet commenced. Only in seven families were weaned babies or older children being given supplements (often Haliborange during the winter) because it was thought they needed 'vitamins'. Several mothers declared robustly that 'you get enough vitamins in what you eat', although some explained the preference for fruit and (in principle) for vegetables by their vitamin content. On the whole they appeared to be thinking in terms only of vitamin C, though one mother at least had heard of the dangers of excess vitamin D:

> I don't believe in dosing them with vitamins. Too much vitamin D is harmful. I don't think there is enough advice on things like cod liver oil. My friend just lets her children eat those capsules like sweets.(M8)

The judgement of the health visitors who knew these families on their diets was critical in a significant minority of cases—perhaps one-quarter of the families. Their criticisms typically included such comments as: 'too much carbohydrates', 'too much stodge', 'too many tins, frozen pies', 'quick meals', 'never in long enough to cook', 'convenience foods', 'baker's vans'. One health visitor tried, not unsympathetically, to explain it thus:

> Families on social security, they have this huge dog with a litter of puppies and don't think twice about spending the money on that. And they were the first to have coloured TVs. We would start at the bottom, spending money on food, and work up. They know they will never work up, so they start at the top.

Our impression in the majority of cases where diets were obviously poor, however, was of inefficiency in spending money rather than a system of values which gave food low priority—an inefficiency largely created by the circumstances of the women's lives, and by commercial pressures. There were only two cases in the sample of children with clinically identified conditions attributed to nutritional deficiency—a girl of three and a girl of four with iron-deficiency anaemia. There may have been others whose illnesses were due to faulty nutrition, particularly among the younger infants, but in the absence of firm clinical attributions we are not able to make this judgement. In general, we have to add that the impression given by the majority of the children was that they were well-developed and well-nourished. As noted earlier, it appears likely from their histories that many more of their mothers were, in fact, ill-nourished as children in the 1950s.

References

[1] Douglas, J. W. B. (1950), 'The extent of breast feeding in Great Britain in 1946', *J. Obstet. Gynaec. Br. Emp.*, **57**, 336.

[2] Davie, R., Butler, N. and Goldstein, H. (1972), *From Birth to Seven: the Second Report of the National Child Development Study (1958 Cohort)*, London: Longman.

[3] Thompson, Barbara (1954), 'Antenatal Attitudes and Infant Feeding Practice', unpublished.

13 Lay Remedies and Lay Referral

One of the questions asked of both grandmothers and mothers was 'Have you got any home remedies that you think are good, especially for children?', followed up by 'Do you ever get anything from the chemist?' and 'Can you remember what your mother's favourite remedies were?' We also asked the mothers what non-prescribed medicines they kept in the house, and of course we recorded exactly what the mother said that the children were given for any illness during the six months, or what home remedies they tried for any of the children's symptoms. The aim was to obtain, from both generations, an account of their beliefs concerning lay remedies or proprietory medicines, and to record the actual use of these for the children as completely as possible.

We thought that this topic might have some historical interest, as far as the grandmother generation was concerned, and we also wished to see whether our families' practices conformed with the pattern generally reported in the literature. It has, of course, commonly been shown that the non-prescribed drugs and remedies which people take far outnumber those they receive from their doctors.[1]

Lay Remedies—the Grandmothers

Most of our grandmothers did offer some account of lay remedies—one great-grandmother who was interviewed was especially informative—though six refused to name any at all, saying they 'didn't believe in them', or that 'it's not safe to use anything except from the doctor'.

All those that were mentioned are listed in Table 13.1, simply for their interest, and because the list provides an indication of the sort of complaint that might be considered suitable for lay treatment. It is obvious that certain remedies were very popular. On the whole, however, there was less enthusiasm for folk remedies and proprietory medicines than we had expected. The women were often describing the 'cures' that their mothers had used, or that they themselves used when their children were small, and though they still believed that these were 'good', they usually hastened to add that scientific

Table 13.1 Grandmothers' lay remedies, especially but not exclusively for children

Condition	Remedy	
	(Numbers indicate the number of women mentioning this remedy, if more than one)	
Colds, flu, sore throat, cough, sore chest	Cough mixture made up by chemist (3)	Balls of butter and sugar
	'Benylin' (5)	Gruel
	'Famel Syrup'	Butter rubbed on nose
	'Beecham's Powders'	Acid drops
	Aspirin (7)	An orange every day
	Camphorated oil or camphor block (4)	'Ackycacky wine' or 'glycerine and apicee' (ipececuana)
	'Vick' (9)	Mustard baths
	Wintergreen	Inhalation of steam
	Saltwater gargle (7)	Hot baths with 'Dettol'
	Toddy—whisky, hot water and sugar (12)	Flannel round the neck (2)
	Lemon and honey (4)	'A sweaty sock round your throat'
	Honey and hot milk and sugar	A sock full of hot salt round the neck (5)
	Glycerine and something sweet	
	Hot milk and syrup	
	Hot Iron Brew (soft drink) and spice	
	Honey and blackcurrant	
Sore ears	Warm olive oil (6)	Almond oil (2)
	'Salt on a shovel at the fire, put it in a woollen sock and put it at your ear'	
Teething	Aspirin (4)	Gripe-water (2)
	Liquid paracetamol (2)	Toddy (2)

Rheumatic pains	Embrocation Chemist's own ointment	'Ballydonny' plaster
Stomach upsets	Boiled water (3) 'Andrews Liver Salts' 'Bisodol'	Dry toast Castor Oil Cornflour and cinnamon
Constipation	'Syrup of Figs' (5) Castor oil	An orange Soap suppositories
Boils, splinters	Kaolin poultice Soap and sugar poultice	Hot lint Bottle full of steam
Sores and cuts	Iodine ointment Zinc and castor oil cream (2) 'Germoline' Bread poultice	Bread and soap poultice Butter Cabbage leaves (2)
Period pains	Footbath of mustard and water	
Burns	Cold water	
Convulsions	Mustard baths	
Rash	Bath with baking soda	
General tonic	'Virol' (2) Yeast and iron tablets – 'Sanatogen wine, with a rich tea biscuit, because it was nourishing' 'A suppie whisky, or port—taken like a medicine, of course, for the iron'	'Syrup of Figs' weekly
'Beasties in the heid'	Paraffin	

Table 13.2 Mothers' lay remedies for children

Condition	Remedy (Numbers indicate the number of women mentioning this remedy, if more than one)	
Colds, coughs, sore throats	'Disprin' (usually *Junior* brand emphasised) (22)	'Veno's Cough Mixture'
	'Codeine'	'Anadin'
	'Benylin' (23)	Chemist's cough mixture (6)
	'Vick' (14)	'Beecham's Powders' (2)
	'Askit' powders	Hot blackcurrant drink (2)
	Hot orange drink (2)	Hot milk and honey
	Hot milk and syrup	'Lemsip'
	Honey and lemon (2)	Soft brown sugar and lemon
	Sugar and butter	Hot ale
	Toddy	
Fever	Aspirin, 'Disprin' (10)	'Calpol' (3)
	Whisky toddy 'to take the temperature down'	Sponging down
Stomach upsets, constipation	'Syrup of Figs' (8)	'Milk of Magnesia' (6)
	'Andrews Liver Salts'	'Eno's Fruit Salts' (2)
	'Diphalac'	'Steadman's Powders'
	Senna	Aspirin
	Brown sugar	Oranges
	Boiled water and salt	Mixture advised by chemist
	Very sweet hot milk and water	

Diarrhoea	A chalky mixture	White of egg and milk
Earache	Olive oil (5)	Drops from chemist
Headache	Aspirin (4)	'Anadin'
	'Codis' (2)	
Toothache	'Disprin' (6)	'Codis' (2)
Teething	'Bonjella' (3)	'Disprin' (6)
	'Calpol' (6)	Gripe water (2)
	Liquid paracetamol	Chemist's powders
Rash	'Savlon' (4)	Calomine (2)
	Cream advised by chemist (4)	
Sores and cuts	'Savlon' (5)	'Germolene'
	'TCP' (2)	'Blistese'
	Zinc cream (4)	Antiseptic creams (8)
	Bread poultice	Bread and soap poultice
General tonics	'Sanatogen' (3)	'Virol'
	Tonic from chemist (2)	

medicine now had better cures, and they would always recommend a prescription from the doctor for a child's symptoms *now*. They also had a healthy scepticism about proprietory medicines in general. One said:

> These cold cures that you buy from the chemist, well, the makers are hoping that you've got a lot of imagination!(G17)

And another said of the embrocation she bought for her rheumatism:

> I *think* it does me good. Whether it's psychological or not I don't know. And possibly the massaging helps!(G11)

They presented themselves as having relied on chemists for remedies in the past, though usually not to a very great extent, but it was not necessary now:

> The doctors, well, when we were bairns your folks had to pay . . . the chemist shops, they were a help. You'd ha' bought a lot of that sorta stuff. A lot of the time it was a waste of money, ye ken! . . . but nowadays tablets cuts out a lot of that things.(G24)

One remedy which, as Table 13.1 shows, was extremely popular and which the grandmothers were loathe to acknowledge substitutes for, was the 'toddy':

> It's a very good remedy, a sup o' toddy. Just two drops maybe, a drop of sugar, and some warm water, and give them maybe just a teaspoon, ken. I told my daughter-in-law that but she said, Oh, no, she wouldnae think o' giein' the children alcohol! Well what they got was just a teaspoon. They get a' these things nowadays, drugs and what nowadays, it's no better.(G63)

They described this as given to quite young babies:

> If they were bothered with their teeth I used to gie them a teaspoon o' whisky, and two teaspoons of sugar in it, and some boiled water, when it cools a wee bittie, ken, you just gie it to them through the bottle and they used to get a good night's sleep and they were a' right.(G31)

and it was still a remedy which many of them favoured for themselves, though sometimes not altogether seriously:

> I dinna ken if it would dae much for your caul', but it makes you feel fine!(G39)

Lay Remedies—the Mothers
Although the list of remedies which the mothers were observed to

use, or said that they used (Table 13.2), includes more proprietory medicines than the list of the grandmothers, in general mothers used only a restricted range of lay remedies for their children. Most of their own mothers' remedies had been given up: 'toddies' were mentioned by very few women, and for the most part it was only soothing drinks (milk and syrup, blackcurrant) which were specifically mentioned as being copied from the older generation. Indeed, several mothers explicitly rejected their own mothers' remedies:

> Not these old wives' tales, where you make up this and make up that. I don't believe in that. Just a Junior Disprin.(M14)
> No, I wouldnae use that stuff she used—that malt stuff shoved down your throat, castor oil an' a'. Nose drops, ear drops, you name it, we got it.(M22)

Several women said that in fact they would never use any lay remedy or proprietory medicine for children at all; they said 'I've never bothered with them', or that they would not even give an aspirin except on the orders of their doctor:

> I don't buy stuff, I'd take them to the doctor. There's such a big range of stuff you dinna know what's in it all. I'd only give them what was prescribed.(M65)

One or two added that, since children's prescriptions carried no charge, buying proprietory medicine was an unnecessary expense and, like their mothers, many women had some scepticism about commercial remedies anyway: 'I don't suppose any of them do any good really. It's silly. But you have to try something.' (M64).

From the list it is evident that a few proprietory medicines were very popular indeed. The reasons volunteered for choosing the most popular cough remedy—which some children appeared to consume large amounts of—were that it had been given to the mothers or the children when they had been in hospital, and that it was advertised on TV. Few mothers believed in regular dosing with laxatives, but there were several families in which Syrup of Figs seemed to be used as a general tonic, sometimes because the mothers remembered being given it or the grandmother recommended it:

> If she hurts herself, mum says to give her Syrup of Figs, to get it out of her system.(M28)

Aspirin, as the list demonstrates, was very freely given to children in the majority of families, occasionally over quite long periods. The mothers were commonly very emphatic about the fact that it was *junior* varieties that were given, and gave the impression of believing that this was quite a different drug to 'ordinary' aspirin. With these few possible exceptions, however, the mothers' use of medicines for their children seemed to be sensible. A few mothers were observed to use drugs prescribed for one child for another who appeared to have the same symptoms, but this is probably a common practice within families. Only one (M30) was observed to give a child medicine which was almost certainly inappropriate, giving him a drug prescribed for the grandmother (probably Valium) 'in order to get a good night's sleep'.

Lay Referral

Studies of the way in which people care for their health have, commonly, suggested not only that lay remedies and non-prescribed drugs are a very important feature, but also that lay advice and help seeking may be as important as consultation with doctors. The literature on 'lay referral', especially from the United States, usually indicates that a formal consultation with a doctor is frequently preceded by (and may indeed be replaced by) a complex pattern of consultation with relatives, friends, and perhaps pharmacists.[2]

Both generations were asked whether they often consulted anyone else about their health, or sought advice about whether they should consult a doctor. In the case of the mothers, we noted what had been reported to us during the six-months' survey period, and asked in the final interview whether the mother thought that this pattern of advice seeking was what she usually did. We also asked who it was among their friends, relatives and neighbours that the respondents talked to about their health generally, or about child development or child care.

The grandmothers

In the grandmothers' replies to our questions, there was in fact little trace of an extensive lay referral system in their present lives. One or two mentioned a particular friend, usually someone much older:

> I've a great friend, she's a trained nurse and everything, I would be asking her what she thought it was that was wrong with me.(G11)

For the most part, however, the women explained that they might mention their symptoms to someone—perhaps their husband—but this was not really asking for *advice*:

> You begin to wonder, you want somebody, you don't feel you want to bother the doctor but you want somebody else to say, yes, go ahead—sort of distribute the blame if you shouldn't have called him in the first place.(G8)

Only two grandmothers mentioned asking a chemist for advice, one because

> After all, what's a chemist? He's just a doctor that's failed one of his tests!(G30)

The great majority denied that they ever discussed health decisions with anyone. They made up their own minds, and went straight to the doctor: 'that's what he's there for'. A few of the women (who were likely to be those in poor health) expressed some feeling of isolation and lack of anybody to talk to about their symptoms:

> [Do you discuss things with your neighbours or friends?] No—why would you want to bother them wi' your health? Naebody's interested in anybody nowadays, are they? Everybody's too much for themselves.(G32)

The mothers

The mothers, as might be expected in a group with young children, described more advice seeking. A few said that they discussed their children's health and development with friends who had children of the same age, or 'some of the mothers at the school', but they were more likely to mention sisters, sisters-in-law, aunts and cousins. Specific advice about symptoms might be asked, in particular, of relatives, friends or neighbours who had some nursing training (or in one case 'a neighbour who is training to be a vet') or who were older and seen as wise and experienced: when M63's child fell, putting his teeth through his lower lip

> I went straight next door and asked Jenny [an old lady who had herself had six children] whether she thought it needed a stitch.(M63)

Similarly, when M70's child seemed ill, her sister, an auxiliary nurse, brought a thermometer to take his temperature before they decided to consult a doctor.

Mothers were particularly likely to run for advice in situations where they said they 'panicked', i.e. accidents, especially if blood was involved, or sudden emergencies. For instance, when her two-year-old daughter fell on the steps M18 ran with her to a neighbour up the road who, she said, was very calm and experienced and good in an emergency:

> ... just, well, wise. She told me not to panic but stay with her a minute and see how E. was, whether she became sleepy or not.(M18)

When a child had an accident, several mothers telephoned their

husbands at work and they came home immediately. M27 was one of
these, and she expressed clearly the special need for support of young
mothers when their own child appears to suffer an emergency: a
baby had been attacked by a puppy and

> ...his face and arms were pouring with blood...I panicked, I
> maybe could have dealt with anybody else's and got them cleaned
> up, but not when it's your own.(M27)

The husband's place in general as an adviser or arbiter of the children's health care varied, as might be expected, depending upon the
couple's individual characters, the nature of the marriage relationship, and the amount of time the husband spent at home.
A characteristic comment was:

> He mostly leaves it up to me. He doesn't like hospitals or doctors
> very much, he's just that type of person, just hates anything to do
> with hospitals or doctors or injections. He always says, you know,
> if the children are ill, Oh, you should call a doctor up here, that's
> what they're there for, they should be brought up here.(M8)

Many husbands were similarly presented (and presented themselves,
if they happened to be there during interviews) as 'bad' patients for
their own illnesses. Where the children were concerned, however,
their wives very often involved them in decisions about service-use,
sometimes waiting until a husband came home in order to have his
support that a doctor was required. In one or two families where the
husband was unemployed and the wife working it was in fact the
husband who had taken the initiative about service-use.
Although a few grandfathers were reported to have been active in
giving advice about the health of their own children or their grandchildren, in general the involvement of husbands seemed to be more
characteristic of the younger generation. The young mothers also
differed from the grandmothers in reporting more use of chemists
for advice (although the grandmothers had of course said that they
did this when their children were young). Twenty-five of the
mothers, or nearly half, said that they would consult a chemist for
some symptoms, or if they were unsure about whether a doctor was
necessary:

> The chemist's awfu' good. He seems to ken as much as the
> doctor.(M27)
> He's very good, most chemists will give advice if you ask.(M63)
> I've got a very good chemist and he advises me. He's been here a
> long time and knows everyone.(M56)

and during the survey period chemists were consulted about many
incidents, principally burns, cuts and rashes.

In general, it appeared that our mothers did make some use of a lay referral system, though it consisted largely of people thought to have special knowledge, rather than being an extensive network of consultation among neighbours and friends. There was, however, a minority of women—about 10 per cent—who insisted that they never asked advice of anyone, or that though they might listen to advice from various sources they would weigh it up themselves and always make their own decisions. This group were confident about their own capability:

> I think I would always have the common sense to do something about it myself.(M32)

and expressed themelves very independently:

> I like to dee a'thing mysel'. I dinna like naebody else's opinions, I like to get my own and ging by what I think.(M36)
> I don't ask advice from anyone if I can help it. I usually try and work things out for myself. I've taken my own approach.(M5)

References
[1] Cartwright, A. and Dunnell, K. (1972), *Medicine Prescribers, Takers and Hoarders*, London: Routledge and Kegan Paul.

[2] e.g. Friedson, E. (1960), *Patients' Views of Medical Practice*, New York: Russell Sage Foundation; (1970), *Profession of Medicine*, New York: Dodd, Mead and Co.
Twaddle, A. (1969), 'Health decisions and sick role variations', *J. of Health and Social Behaviour*, **10**, 105.

14 Attitudes to Medicine, Doctors and Health Services

Attitudes to medicine as an institution and to doctors and other providers of health services, and reactions to the organisation of these services, are of course one set of intervening variables between the concepts of health and sickness which were discussed in chapter 4 and the use of services, in different contexts, which has been documented in the subsequent chapters. As these chapters have shown, attitudes to medicine and doctors are not the only mediating influence: economic conditions, the environment, practical contingencies, and life circumstances all have their place in explaining the patterns of association between any particular concept of illness and the actions that are taken. Nor are attitudes to doctors a *determinant* of help-seeking behaviour, for of course the process is interactive. Experiences in help seeking and perceptions of the available services in turn create or reinforce the attitudes to doctors, and to the concept of health, on which further help seeking may depend.

For these reasons, the significance of the women's attitudes to service-providers is not altogether easy to determine. Empirically, it was equally found that the analysis was complex. It was noted previously that attitudes to health and illness were not necessarily consistent, logical or easily described on single dimensions. This applied even more strongly to attitudes to doctors and health services, which (as one might expect) were highly contingent. They might vary over time, relate to one group of service-providers but not others, or be crucially influenced by salient events and specific to individual professionals. Nevertheless, it was obvious that, in general, attitudes to health services *did* differ markedly between the generations, and that this difference was important in explaining health behaviour.

The topic is considered under four headings: attitudes to medicine, relationships with doctors, views on the organisation of primary care, and attitudes to other services (principally health visiting). The method of deriving attitudes to medicine and to doctors was in each case to form, from the interview transcripts, as exhaustive as possible a list of dichotomies in attitude. Examples are, for medicine, belief in/distrust of scientific medicine, active/passive towards treatment, fear/trust, optimistic/pessimistic about cure, and many others; for doctors, grateful/critical, deferential/belligerent, liking for impersonal professional/'family doctor', and so on. All phrases, comments, answers to questions or stories recounted which were relevant to these topics were then extracted from the transcripts and interview notes, and a cumulative picture built up of the different sets of attitudes in each generation.

Attitudes to Medicine

Many of the grandmothers paid lip-service to the marvels of modern scientific medicine:

> Look at the things they dee for heart-attack patients now! They can dee wonders for them. Before my time, I mean, fit tablets was there really? They could even pit in a pacer an' a'thing now. It's marvellous, really, how they think up things like that!(G40)

They rarely gave the impression, however, of feeling that these advances applied to them personally. They acknowledged that drugs, in particular, were more effective nowadays, and commonly asked for antibiotics, for instance, to clear infections. On the whole, however, despite the theoretical admiration for medical science (much fuelled by television programmes) they often preferred, for themselves, to fall back upon 'mind over matter' models of cure. These may obviously be associated with the similar models of cause described in chapter 4. One woman described how, by determination alone, she had recovered from what appeared to be a quite severe stroke. Several explained non-compliance with medical regimens by claiming that strength of mind was more effective than drug therapy:

> There's lots of times I've went to the doctor and I've taken the first two tablets—I never took the rest—'Oh, I'll manage!' And I *have* mended. I mean, in my own faith.(G33)

The younger generation, as might be expected, took modern scientific medicine much more for granted. For them, its benefits *should* be available. They said things like: 'I don't want him to just examine her. I'd like him to put her to the hospital for a cardiograph' (M6); 'The bedside manner is OK but that's no good if they can't cure you' (M39); 'I aye say, if there's onything *really* serious crops up, the doctors nowadays, they've a' the equipment and a'thing, nothing can really go wrong.' (M16) Indeed, life without the benefits of medical science was unthinkable:

> I'm a healthy person really. What I have can be cleared up in a

couple of weeks with a course. But I dread to think what would
happen if I was stuck on an island or something. Piles, for
example—I'd be up the wall. And what would a chill on the kid-
neys turn into if you wasn't getting a course of penicillin to put it
awa'?(M12)

A belief in the efficacy of medicine did not necessarily mean, however, that the young women knew how to obtain its benefits. Indeed,
their higher expectations of what medicine ought to do sometimes
led to greater frustration, and this in turn might eventually produce
apathy and passivity.

Both older and younger women looked for palliation rather than
cure of chronic conditions. When asked, 'Do you think they're
making advances with diseases like yours?' one of the grandmothers
replied:

Well, I've niver actually thought about it in that way. Because
what I've been given any time, that always helps me. I know it
helps me. Or else I wouldn't be able to go out and work.(G30)

There was thus a great deal of fatalism, rather than optimism and
hope, about more serious conditions, and non-compliance with
medical advice or lack of consultation could be explained by 'not
wasting people's time' as well as by 'strength of character':

I was going back and fore to the clinic . . . but they said they could
never get my blood up to 100 per cent . . . I says, well, if that's it I
don't see any sense of coming back. Because it was wastin' their
time when they could have somebody else. There's no sense of
clutterin' up a place when there's no need for it.(G30)

Of course, fear and fatalism about outcomes might also be
offered—as might be expected, among the older rather than the
younger women—as reasons for not making use of medical services.
Most of the older women said that cervical smear tests were an
excellent thing, but a high proportion produced various reasons for
never having had one. Some women consulted immediately about
particularly frightening symptoms (lumps in the breast, or pains
suggestive of heart disease), but others said that they would prefer
'not to know':

You know, if I discovered a lump I would just hold on to it—I
wouldnae say 'Oh yes, go ahead and operate'—I think I would
hold on to it, until, probably it was too late.(G29)

At the extreme, this passivity and fatalism could include a remarkable lack of curiosity. Examples among the younger women are one
who could not name her husband's quite severe hereditary disease,

or one who never inquired about the cause of a child's convulsions. Among the older women, there was one who, over sixteen years, had not inquired whether a sterilisation operation had involved a hysterectomy: 'She never really telt me, but I've never been back to the doctor to find out either', and another who said:

> When the gynaecologist says, 'Do you want to ask me onything about the operation?' I says, 'No, I dinna want to ken!'(G19)

This most fearful and passive group of women were likely to dread medical examinations and express worries about 'interference with nature', They consistently talked of illness as 'bad luck' or 'just one o' that things that happens', and did not appear to feel that medicine could have much effect upon the essentially haphazard and inevitable nature of disease.

Attitudes to Doctors

For both those who were actively favourable to medicine and those who were passive and fatalistic, the most common set of attitudes among the older generation towards doctors included trust, gratitude, and a liking for the 'family doctor' relationship. Talking of the past, they were proud to tell many stories of the 'great men'—well-known family doctors, or important consultants—whom they had known. One displayed amazed gratitude because 'the Professor' used to give her son five shillings when he saw him at the clinic:

> That a man o' his profession should *think*, even, o' givin' W. such a thing!(G1)

Another was enthusiastic about the way that

> *Even* the doctors an' that, or the surgeons, will sit an' talk to you—that Professor M., the way he jist sat an' chatted to you about things to try and find out what was bothering me.(G11)

and another recounted how

> It wis Dr S. this last time, he says, 'I've seen you before' an' I says, 'Aye, seventeen, well, eighteen years ago', I says, 'but you've been in my hoose an' a''. He says, 'That's right', he says, 'eighteen years ago—dinna let on wur age! I'm an aul' man!' But Dr S., he's a specialist, he's very nice.(G13)

They also had many stories of what they saw as consideration, kindness, and devoted service from family doctors of the past:

> But Dr B., he couldn't have been better—he came up, we didn't have very much at the time, you know, the wages were little and

we had the two kids, I wasnae workin', an' he came up the next morning, you know, after [the child] had died, and said that he was very sorry and he shook hands with my husband and he shook hands with me, and you know—I felt something in my hand, and he just said goodbye and he went away and when I looked he had given me £2. And he just—went away... he was really excellent.(G29)

Almost unanimously this generation saw the days of the family doctor as, regrettably, past. Doctors being 'busier', having more patients, or the present-day 'abuse' of the service by patients who 'turn to the doctor for the least little thing', were all blamed for the impersonality of services now:

The family doctor has lost contact with the patients. The family doctor days are finished, of course... we're livin' in a different time. But long ago you felt, when the doctor came in, you could talk to him. He took time to listen. And I don't feel like that now... but nowadays, you see, they reckon that all the doctors in the practice are your doctor.(G37)

The women were telling stories of the past, of course, and there seemed to be some tendency to dramatise or exaggerate—whether positively or negatively—the events of long ago. The 'horror' stories of neglect and misdiagnosis, though very much less frequent than the laudatory tales, were equally emphatic. Whether all, or many, of these women actually had the sort of relationship with their doctor that they described must remain open: indeed, one at least believed that there was a greater distance between doctor and patient in the past:

You can speak to them better now—the older type of doctor, you just said what you had to say and you couldnae say anything more.

and ascribed a mythical view of the doctor–patient relationship to the media:

I think there's too much of what you see in TV. You know, they know everybody by their first name, an' sittin' having a news [gossip] for hours wi' them—I think there's a lot of that on the TV, the American idea. A lot of folk think that we should be like that. But, I mean, the doctor has a lot to see and a lot to do... I feel they couldn't really have a personal touch.(G25)

The younger generation were more varied in their descriptions of the ideal doctor–patient relationship. A proportion, often those who had known the same doctor since childhood, were similar to their mothers in thinking that the presence or absence of a family doctor relationship was important: they liked someone who knew them by their first name, whom they found it easier to speak to.

The majority, however, said that they did not care greatly about which doctor they saw in a practice (as long as it was not particular individuals whom they disliked), or that they might choose to see different doctors for different purposes. Many of them saw doctors as interchangeable:

> They all have the same qualifications, after all.(M18)
> It's a good idea to be able to pick which one you want.(M70)

and a few specifically rejected the family doctor model:

> Oh, I wouldn't like that. You don't want someone knowing all about you. I just want a doctor for whatever I want him for . . . I just want him to say what it is and give you the stuff or whatever.(M64)

Associated with the older generation's liking for the family doctor were characteristic attitudes of deference, gratitude, and a remarkable trust. The symbol of the doctor as the one on whose shoulders reponsibility falls, the professional whose mere presence is crucial, no matter what he may actually do, was vividly explained by several respondents, of whom these are typical:

> If he says [the child] is all right, he's all right. It doesn't matter if he's the same after the doctor goes away, as long as the doctor's been and said it's all right.(G22)
> I phoned the doctor an' he says, 'I'm not coming out' he says, 'there's nothing I can do for him' [the patient was terminally ill]. Well, Rab just felt then, he's given me up. Even if he'd come and given him an aspirin . . . Rab would have been none the wiser, but he'd just have felt, well, the doctor's come.(G25)

Even at the present time, many of the older women rarely appeared to question diagnosis or the nature or objective of treatment, simply accepting what was said to them (though not necessarily, as already noted, complying with it). One woman did express clearly the view that the change from deference to a questioning attitude was a temporal one, rather than distinguishing between the generations, but she was representative of only a small minority:

> At one time, whatever they said I sorta hung onto, ken, but now I believe him, but at the same time I've got this 'Och, I dinna think he could be right', sorta thing. It's maybe just that I'm getting older, ken . . . but when you're in the hospital an' a doctor come to you, at one time you just sorta lie there—'God, fit's comin' next?'—ken. But now, I would hae nae hesitation in sayin' to the doctor, 'Why are ye deein' this?' I would ask the doctor.(G30)

This scepticism was very mild compared with that expressed by a group of the younger generation. Amongst these mothers, there was little evidence of the doctor being an idealised figure—one woman's ironic description was more typical:

> There's this thing about doctors, you're scared of wasting their time. They're like gods, sometimes—it's silly, I don't know why. It's their job, they're paid to see patients. I've seen me going down one week with one of them and then again the next week with the next, and I think—Oh, no, they'll say not me again.(M70)

Most mothers had a non-deferential, critical way of speaking of what they saw as poor doctoring, and they rarely gave the impression, common among the grandmothers, of being surprised and horrified if they thought that an error had been made. A proportion of them presented themselves as aggressive towards service-providers:

> The receptionist asked if it was worth the GP calling and I said yes, it's bloody worth him calling!(M13)

or insistent that services must be arranged to suit their own circumstances: one mother's account of her interaction with doctors was:

> He said, 'Are you sure it's gallstones?' I said 'Of course I'm sure, you just look at the notes, there's X-rays and everything.' . . . after I got to the hospital the doctor came round and looked at me and said 'You look all right, we'll keep you in for a day or two'. . . I said, 'Oh, no, I'm not walking out of here, now I've come I want it seen to!' I said, 'The quicker the blooming better, I've lain here waiting for two days already.'(M68)

If they believed that the service was faulty, they were prepared to be belligerent about demanding what they wanted, without deference towards doctors:

> He wasn't going to come out and I went mad. I said I would go for the police doctor.(M17)
> Why should I hae to put up wi' that? You shouldna have to put up wi' anything like that. Nae from him or anyone else.(M5)
> He said I could have it done privately. He must have been touting for trade.(M34)

These women were likely to have firm ideas about treatment, and to present themselves as having made their wishes clear:

> He was a bit sharp, said it was just a rash, he didn't know what it was. He said try some camomile lotion. I said, 'Do I buy it from the chemists?' And he said, 'Oh, well, here's a prescription' . . . I'm not cowed by doctors.(M64)

It has, of course, been shown in other studies that though 'in the recounting of an encounter between the teller/patient and the doctor, the former is portrayed as playing a very active part', in actuality 'the patient tends to be acquiescent, speaking more quietly than the doctor, in response to the doctor, and rarely contradicting the doctor outright'.[1] Stimson and Webb suggest that the patient uses the story as a vehicle for making herself rational and sensible, and to redress the inequalities between patient and doctor. This group of the younger generation certainly chose to present themselves as not meekly accepting poor service in a fatalistic way. Whether or not they did make overt demands as they said, they certainly actively exercised choice and control, using the facilities available—more than one general practitioner, clinics, the children's hospital—in a 'supermarket' manner, choosing what they saw as the 'best buy' for a particular occasion.

Another group of the younger generation, however, were equally critical but much more passive. Typically, these women talked of their doctors very impersonally, and they registered disapproval simply by not keeping appointments, or refusing to say very much during consultations. Some of them tended to blame the services for the misfortunes that befell them, and others indicated that they felt that they themselves were being judged unfavourably by service-providers:

I'm getting into trouble for not taking him for his injections.
The hospital usually seem to *blame* you for what's happened.(M27)

Their accounts were full of descriptions of what they 'felt like saying' to doctors or other health-service personnel, but never in fact claimed that they did say. Even in a case where a doctor's receptionist had refused to give the result of a pregnancy test, and the mother said that she 'felt like saying this is my third! I want to know!' (M38), she did not actually claim to have said it.

Obviously these women felt that their interaction with service-providers was often unsatisfactory, and they were particularly dependent upon their general practitioners, for unlike the more positive and active mothers they did not have the confidence to approach different services, and their sense of powerlessness prevented them from taking steps to alter the situation, for instance by changing their doctor.

Opinions of Service Structures
Whether or not a respondent had positive attitudes to medicine in the

abstract, and whether or not she thought highly of doctors, she might of course have views on the actual services available to her which were highly dependent on her present experience and perceived needs. She might be, in general, very favourable towards doctors as a group but dislike the one she was in contact with; she might believe that medicine was advancing marvellously but that the particular services in her own area were poor. We present here a description of those features of the organisation of medical services which were of most importance to the women of each generation.

The young women, as might be expected, took the National Health Service completely for granted. Their mothers, on the other hand, were apt to be enthusiastic about it, in principle:

> ...you see, the poor people that are ill, 'Oh, we canna get the doctor cos we hinna money to pey the bill'—it's like gaun back to the cave ages. Do you nae think so? ... ha'in to hesitate to bring in a doctor, that's like goin' back decades, that. No—I think the Health Service is the finest thing that ever happened in this country.(G40)

On the other hand, as already indicated, the majority of the older generation thought that the 'family doctor' service had in fact deteriorated sadly, and that there were aspects of the organisation of services that were not only less pleasant, in their eyes, but also less efficient:

> Say you've got one doctor, and then the next time you go you get a completely different doctor. And then they don't know your illness, they've to go and get your records... and when they come to the house they never bring their records. They never have the records with them. You know, before, they used to look up and see things. Now, when they come in they ask *you* what's wrong...we wouldnae call them in if we knew whit wis wrong!(G32)

Despite their many criticisms of what they saw as a more impersonal service, however, the older women were very reluctant to change from one doctor to another. A new doctor, they argued very logically, might well mean an even more impersonal relationship: G30 agreed that she *had* thought of changing her doctor, but she decided not to 'lift her cards' because, after all, 'They've *got* everything, they ken oor lives mair or less.'

For the young mothers, the distinguishing feature of good or bad medical practice was willingness to make house-calls. A 'good' doctor was one who came promptly. 'If I phone back of nine she's here by ten. I *never* have to wait', and a 'bad' doctor was one who was 'not that ready to come in', or took too long to arrive. For the grandmothers, making quick and ready house-calls was similarly the mark of a 'good' doctor, but either their demands were lower, or there was in fact less conflict in their case about house-calls, for a much smaller proportion mentioned reluctance to come to their house. Indeed, one or two criticised because the doctor 'only comes when he's called', suggesting that they expected the doctor to 'drop in' unsummoned. It may well be, of course, that more conflict is inevitable for the mothers of young children, with all their problems of deciding when a child is 'really' ill.

Other aspects of service mentioned by almost all mothers were difficulties about getting quick appointments at the surgery, or surgeries being difficult to reach or having inconvenient hours. In part, these service difficulties were due to the inevitable practical difficulties of young families, especially those (the majority) without telephones or cars, and to some maldistribution of medical practices, with few in the large housing estates:

> ...obviously, a bad case of sickness and diarrhoea, it's very difficult—it takes an hour to get there! If it's only one and you can get a babysitter for the other two it's not so bad, and if you can get a taxi of course it doesnae take that long. But you can't always afford a taxi.(M8)

In part, however, it must be noted that many of the families, both older and younger, caused their own problems by their pattern of service-use—remaining registered with doctors at a considerable distance from their homes, or having different members of the family registered with different practices. It was quite common for husband and wife, in the younger generation, to remain registered with the separate doctors they had had before marriage, and a third doctor known to be 'good with children' might have been chosen for the children.

During the survey period there were some attempts by doctors to rationalise their practices by suggesting (or in two cases insisting) that all the family register with the same practice, or change to one more geographically convenient. This caused some complaint in the younger generation, who did not see why it was necessary to have a 'family' doctor, and in the older generation if it meant a new doctor in the place of one they had known for many years. On the other hand, many doctors gave very willing service to families living an inconvenient distance from their practices. In general, however, it is obvious that if considerable distances were involved, the irritation of doctors called frequently to the home—perhaps for conditions which turned out to be trivial—might be reinforced.

The structure of services was also a point of criticism in the younger generation, with some problems about the relative functions of the general practitioner and the child clinic, where a doctor might offer assessment and advice but not treatment.

> If you go to your own doctor he tells you to go to the clinic, they tell you to go to your own doctor—it's a vicious circle.(M37)

Instead of routine willingness to call, for a greater proportion of the grandmothers delay in getting appointments or difficulty in getting to the surgery were important features of the doctor's service. This matched very well a marked difference between the generations in the reported principles on which they based their service-use, with 'I'd always get the doctor. That's what they're there for' (M68) being more typical of mothers, and 'To call a doctor to the house I'd have to be really ill . . . I think he's got enough to do without having to trail out' (G17) more typical of the older generation. Another marked difference was that almost all mothers saw appointments systems as a favourable feature of general practice organisation, while quite a high proportion of the older generation preferred the older system of simply going to the doctor's surgery and waiting their turn:

> Just see him the old way, to me wis the best . . . you just went doon an' waited your turn, it disna' matter how long you waited your turn.(G15)

In some ways, however, the model of good service held by the grandmothers displayed higher expectations than that of the mothers. The mothers might expect efficient responses to their demands, but many grandmothers (and only a few mothers) talked at length of the exceptional and very personal service they saw as their ideal, involving very frequent calls, and a considerable amount of the doctor's time; often, these referred very specifically to the past. A long story of a child's pneumonia is perhaps typical, ending:

> He attended that bairn, morning an' night, morning an' night . . . an' he telt me if he'd pit her away to hospital, he says, 'But I kent, if I pit her awa' it would hae been a worry for you'—I'd only a kitchen and bedroom then, ken. Six o' us bade there. An' he bathed her oot o' a basin, an' sponged her a' doon, an' dried her—an' he did the same til her doll—the verra same til her doll. He wis verra good.(G15)

The amount of time the doctor had to spare for a consultation was a salient feature of service for both generations. Grandmothers, particularly, defined a 'good' doctor as one who could offer his time, and a 'bad' doctor as one who 'has the prescription written out before you've ever spoken' (G2), but though these comments were extremely frequent they were very often combined with excuses and sympathy for the doctor:

> They just don't seem to have the time they used to have years and years ago—but I think it's not the doctors' fault, they're pressured.(G22)
> I know doctors are overworked, and they work long hours, but so does a lot of other people—to me, a doctor's paperwork now.(G37)

Both mothers and grandmothers blamed doctors' receptionists for what they saw as service failures, and (particularly the mothers) thought that it would be more efficient if the doctor would speak to the patient personally on the telephone:

> The doctor should come to the phone, the receptionists shouldn't be giving you what to do about medical things.(M56)

The receptionist's function of protecting the doctor from 'abusing' patients, however, was more often mentioned by older women:

> [after a story of difficulty in getting an appointment] I think once you get past the receptionist you're a' right—*If* you get past—I mean, she's looking after the doctor's interests—there was that instance . . . but I dinna suppose they want to overbook the doctor, too much work for him.(G25)

It is notable that administrative features of the NHS were very rarely mentioned by either group of women. Complaints about difficulty in getting drugs were not common (rather the reverse: 'too many tablets') and the right of the general practitioner to act as gate-keeper for referral to specialist or hospital services was almost never questioned. Quasi-medical services such as sickness certification for employment purposes or 'lines' for housing were taken for granted and seen as unproblematic. Costs were mentioned only a few times: two respondents thought that they paid 'too much' for the NHS (through their National Insurance) and two of the older women suggested that there might be better service if payment were direct.

Health Visitors
In the same way as with doctors, the women's attitudes to their health visitors were not necessarily consistent. They might change quite radically, depending on particular incidents or the personality of particular nurses. The grandmothers' remembered experience of

health-visiting services varied greatly; a few recalled particular health visitors with gratitude and affection, a few had disliked them, some had had little experience, and most said routinely that the service was 'a good thing'.

Of the mothers, about a fifth expressed wholly negative views, implying that they saw the service as interference or, as several said, 'just a waste of time'. The main objection which these women had was of being told what to do, especially (as noted in Chapter 12) in relation to infant feeding, by women who had no family of their own:

> My last health visitor had no children of her own, so I don't know how she would know. They maybe get trained, but I don't think it's the same as having a baby and doing it.(M14)

On the other hand, at least two-fifths could be called enthusiastic about the service. They mentioned particularly how much they had appreciated the health visitor's help when their children were babies, especially the first, when they might have been lonely and depressed. The health visitor was someone who 'didn't take sides', and so was a more impartial adviser than family members. Several of the women who expressed favourable views said that in fact they would have liked more frequent visiting, especially when they had young babies.

We thought it of interest to explore the women's concept of what the function of the health visitor was, whether they themselves felt they needed the service or not. Those with a good relationship with their health visitor saw her as a valued friend, making comments such as:

> She's a person that if you've any problems with your children she's there to tell about it, to help you with them. [This mother added that this was better than] taking out your depression on the children or talking to the neighbours.(M25)
> If something is troubling you, that's really troubling your health as well, that's their job as well. The more they know about the family, the better idea they get to what's wrong.(M41)
> If I was bothered about anything...I'd just pick up the phone...they would come right down. Just into their cars and come right down, they're good like that.(M40)

This last mother, however, had many long-term problems involving conflict with health services, with which it had not seemed that the health visitor had been able to help. Obviously, where there is con-flict between doctor and patient, the health visitor is placed in a very difficult position. There were other mothers who appeared to be using their health visitors very much as social workers, expecting not only support but practical assistance (especially over housing). One mother said that health visitors were 'better than your social workers!' and another actually called her health visitor 'my social worker from the GP'.

It was, however, very notable that a high proportion of our respondents volunteered the view that one of the functions of the health visitor—perhaps the major one—was to police child neglect or child abuse. Those who felt they had not needed advice or help themselves often added that, nevertheless, the service was essential: one mother described health visitors as '. . . interfering in some ways, but they find out a lot of child battering that way'. Others described the health visitor's function as:

> . . . to see they weren't being starved. They wouldn't let you starve them.(M23)
> . . . to see your house is clean and tidy for a baby to be in—if you had any family problems I suppose they would report it.(M24)

In some cases this view was extended to child health clinics also: M30 said that she used to attend '. . . just to let them see they weren't being battered—they're just there to see you treat them OK'. This recurrent theme of the possibility of being suspected of 'battering' was noted before in connection with accidents. At one of our interviews, a child was found to have had a simple accident resulting in a black eye. The mother's immediate comment was 'It's a good job you're not the health visitor!' Of course, for the great majority of mothers, to whom the idea that their children should be ill-treated was ridiculous, this policing function of the health visitor applied to 'other people', not to them: there appeared to be a perhaps exaggerated stock of third-hand stories of the amount of child abuse that was current. For the minority of mothers who had, for some reason, felt that their child care was being criticised by health visitors, however, this defensiveness about the suspicion of abuse was an obvious cause of conflict.

Child Health Clinics and School Health Services

The grandmothers' experience of child health clinics did not, in most cases, seem to us to be remembered or recounted with any great accuracy. Some did remember that they had found clinics useful, but the majority said that they had used their own GPs for immunisations and routine baby care, and made remarks such as· 'I didnae bother with the clinic' (G13), or 'I must admit I wisnae all that great on it.' (G17) It seems likely that this group had, in fact, not been very frequent attenders at clinics. They realised that this was not very 'approved' behaviour, and offered a variety of excuses:

> And there was a bairn there had a chickenpox and I walked in wi'
> my bairn—I walked out again. 'Cos that was actually infectious
> diseases, was it? I didnae go back again.(G4)
> To get them weighed I used to ging to the chemist—ken, they used
> to have a basket. You went up to the clinic, you'd just hae washed
> and dressed them to take to the clinic, you had to tak' a'thing off
> again—just to get them weighed . . . it was just a pandemonium
> so—they got weighed in the chemist.(G12)

One other quotation perhaps summarises the not always consistent
mixture of conventional approval with memories of their own
defaulting:

> Clinics, yes, I *think* I went ower to the clinic wi' B. and C.—I did-
> nae ging an awfu' lot back and forwards to the clinic . . . I didnae
> really *need* to ging to a clinic for advice or onything like that,
> because I hid my mother at my back, ken? . . . But, oh, I think the
> clinics are a good thing. Especially for any that's maybe naebody
> at their back and naebody that can help. An' I aye found them
> awfu' nice. It *is* a good thing, the clinic.(G6)

The mothers, according to the records and their own accounts, were
more frequent clinic attenders, especially when their babies were
young or for the first child. For most mothers, attendance became
rarer with second and subsequent children. For the most part, however, the mothers, like the grandmothers, gave conventionally
approving rather than enthusiastic responses, saying that clinics were
'very helpful', 'reassuring', they 'quite liked going', 'didn't have
much to ask about but if you did they were very helpful', it was
better than 'bothering your doctor for something unnecessary' or
'quite convenient for children with minor ailments, without having
to make an appointment with the doctor'. A few women also
stressed the social functions of the clinics, especially for new
mothers:

> It's good for a young mother with her first baby, she wants to go
> and show off her baby, meet other mothers.(M13)

Where practices had their own health visitors and their own clinics,
the mothers tended to prefer these, sometimes saying they were
'more friendly'. Others preferred to use their GP for all infant care,
especially if he (or more probably she) was known to be 'a good baby
doctor'. One mother explained that she always went to her own doctor because 'at the clinic they're seeing children every two minutes'
and so never got to know the child (M10). There was also variation,
of course, in the convenience with which the clinics were situated for
particular mothers. In some housing estates the nearest local

authority clinic was an awkward journey distant.

Because of this variety of patterns of service-use and service-provision, it is not easy to make any quantitative assessments of clinic use in the sample. A minority of women said frankly that they had never liked, and never used, clinics; they gave a variety of reasons, such as not wanting immunisation, conflict over infant feeding, dislike of having to undress children unnecessarily (as G12 had said), 'it just seemed a trail for nothing—all uphill, pushing a pram' (M11), or 'I was put off because I thought one or two of the kids weren't as clean as they might be.' (M63) Only one of the mothers was eloquent about her feelings that the service was offered in an insulting way:

> Like there was one day I went up—to give you an example—I went up one day, and there was this lassie sitting there waiting, and you kent that she didnae hae much. She'd a quinie [a girl] and this little baby. An' the woman there says 'I've got some clothes here for the baby' and the lass just sat there and looked at her, ken. And you kent fine she'd hae grabbed them, if she'd taken her through to her room and said til her 'OK, you help yourself out of these claes to what you want for your kiddies', ken . . . and I felt really sorry for her.(M1)

This was followed by a story of M1 herself being offered a pram, and replying indignantly, 'I dinna need your pram, I'm getting a pram.'

Many of the mothers who admitted they had never attended clinics might, however, have obtained the equivalent services from their health visitors and GPs. There were only a few mothers whose non-attendance at clinics definitely represented some apathy or neglect, and these were of course likely to be the same group, all in the 'more disadvantaged' families, whose lack of concern for preventive care had been noted in connection with immunisation.

The *school health services* were remarkable for their lack of salience for our mothers. In most of the relevant cases, it was noted that the mother did accompany the child to school medical examinations. They had very little to say about them, however, typically remarking only that 'it's good to have a check'. In a few cases, sight and hearing problems were picked up at these examinations, but the mothers rarely reported having taken the opportunity to discuss the child's health.

Attitudes to Services and Propensity to Use Them

We have, of course, no independent data on the use of services by the grandmothers, or the use of services by the mothers for themselves.

Some attempt will be made, however, to relate the attitudes to medicine and to doctors which have been described to the propensity of individual women to make use of curative and preventive services.

A scoring of each woman on all the dimensions used in this analysis, and a simple cluster analysis, showed that there were six categories into which they most easily fell. Giving them arbitrary names, they were:

(1) the *active and compliant*, whose views of health and doctors were predominantly positive, optimistic, and co-operative,
(2) The *active and demanding*, not so obedient and trusting, with a positive view of medicine but an aggressive stance towards service-providers,
(3) The *active and critical*, who like the first two appeared to have a sense of control over their own health, but were either positively anti-medicine or very critical of it,
(4) the *passive and deferential*, with a fatalistic view of health but nevertheless trusting, deferential and grateful attitudes to doctors,
(5) the *passive but dissatisfied*, critical and complaining but passive in their reported interactions with service-providers,
(6) the *apathetic*, neither grateful nor critical towards services, and completely pessimistic about medicine and about their own health.

There were examples of each group in both generations. The older generation, however, were more likely to be categorised as *passive and deferential* (one third) or *active and compliant* (one quarter). Their daughters were distributed through all the categories, but the greatest number (one quarter) was in the *passive but dissatisfied* group.

The *reported* principles of service-use (and what evidence was available of actual service-use from the survey period, or from the existence of chronic conditions, etc.) of women in the different categories did suggest that there was some association between these sets of attitudes and propensity to use services, though its nature was different in the two generations. The grandmothers almost all presented themselves as reluctant to seek medical services, and it appeared to be true that they consulted relatively infrequently. Those with the most active and positive views of medicine recounted the greatest use of services.

Among the great majority of the young women, however, attitudes did not appear to affect greatly the willingness to consult. Most of them presented themselves as using services quite frequently, expressing little of their mothers' reluctance, whether or not they were critical of those services. The *active and demanding* or *active and compliant* were, as might be expected, certainly high users of services for their children, in relation to the perceived need. The *active and critical, passive and deferential*, and most of the group who were *passive but dissatisfied*, were equally ready to use curative services (and more likely to perceive more ill health) but not necessarily preventive services.

It was the last group, described as the *apathetic*, who were most likely in both generations to avoid both preventive and curative services, saying, for instance, 'I try to keep away from doctors' or 'I dinna bother.' Despite the fact that their health tended to be poor, they simply did not see health-related activities as of any priority. This is the group which perhaps most nearly fits the stereotype of the 'culture of poverty'. It is therefore important to emphasise how small a minority of women of either generation were found to fall within it in this sample. This small group, as far as the young families was concerned, was entirely among those categorised as 'more disadvantaged'.

References

[1] Stimson, G. and Webb, B. (1975), *Going to See the Doctor*, London: Routledge and Kegan Paul.

15 Mothers and Daughters: Intergenerational Influences

Throughout the discussion of various aspects of health care and health attitudes, the emphasis has so far been on a comparison of the two generations as groups. We have been asking: in what ways are the behaviour and attitudes of the two groups of women similar, and in what way different; are changes due simply to the fact that we are considering groups at different stages of the life cycle, or have there been real temporal changes associated with social change and a different structure of health services?

In this chapter we look more closely at continuities, and at mother–daughter pairs. Despite the evidence from many studies[1] (principally from the United States) that maternal grandmothers are still a primary source of familial assistance in time of illness, the exact ways in which the older generation may influence the actions of their adult children is not a subject which has received much research attention. In the three-generational study of Litman,[2] the younger generation certainly *said* that their parents were the most salient source of health advice and opinions, and there is a conventional common-sense wisdom of 'like mother, like daughter' to which some of the grandmothers in this study similarly subscribed:

> [Talking of lay remedies] . . . just what *my* mother used. Just sort of passes on. And my lot'll pass on what I tell them. Same wi' bringing up their children, they'll just sorta do the things *I* did wi' them, you see.(G23)

Most of these statements sounded more conventional than real, however; in part, they seemed to be another aspect of the appeal to continuity, stability and meaningfulness which had been displayed in the liking for 'heredity' as an explanation for disease.

Service-providers express the same views: the health visitors who were interviewed, for instance, certainly described the grandmothers as the most salient source of lay advice and influence in these particular families. They believed that many child-care practices and lay remedies were passed on through the generations:

Grandmothers are one of our biggest problems. Mums are very receptive to old tips like butter on the nose rather than nasal sprays from the health visitor, because *their* mothers used that!

But, as one health visitor said ruefully, 'How can you tell a great-granny who's brought up ten of her own!' In infant feeding—especially the early feeding of solids, which was one of the practices the health visitors found most difficult to combat—they felt that the grandmothers were especially influential. On this particular subject, there was some evidence that this was partially true. For the most part, however, the influence of the older generation did not appear to be nearly as strong as the health visitors supposed.

Direct Advice and Influence

The topic was approached in various ways. Most directly, each grandmother was asked whether she gave advice to her daughter, what that advice consisted of, and how it was received, and the daughters were asked the equivalent questions. These are, of course, accounts, which have to be compared both with specific beliefs and attitudes, and with behaviour. The interview material was also examined to see whether mothers and daughters expressed similar ideas and beliefs. Finally, during the survey months special note was taken of the extent to which the grandmothers were involved in the children's illness episodes or appeared to be influential in their general management.

It might have been expected that the accounts of mother and daughter would frequently disagree, though each did know, of course, that the other was being interviewed. In fact, when the individual pairs of interviews were compared, there was a remarkable consistency. This is shown in Table 15.1, where the older and

Table 15.1 *Grandmothers' and mothers' accounts of advice-giving compared, number of families*

| | Grandmother's response | | |
Mother's response	Yes, gives advice and it is welcomed	Equivocal	No, never interferes
Yes, grandmother gives advice and it is welcomed	13	3	1
Equivocal	2	3	2
No, never receives or accepts advice	1	1	21

young generations' responses are set against each other, for the 47
pairs in which the grandmother was interviewed.

It can be seen that there were only two families where completely
contradictory accounts were given. The largest group is that where
both mother and daughter agreed that the daughter went her own
way entirely. A smaller group agreed that the older generation's
influence was important. In the remaining pairs, one or both was
equivocal: advice was given or accepted to some extent:

> Yes, they ask, but I think they still please themselves!(G25)
> Oh aye, I listen! I don't say I agree wi' it all, but I listen!(M25)

Most of the older generation said that they had been greatly
influenced by their own mothers, and had always received advice
from them. G40, saying that she did influence her daughter,
explained:

> . . . I think that's how it passes on, 'cos it wis my mother that
> passed it on to me, I used to run to my mother a lot.(G40)

and another grandmother described specific advice of the sort that
was occasionally documented for children's illnesses during the
survey period:

> She'll phone me doon and she'll say, Mum, T.'s got an awful
> caul' . . . she's got croup, she's been sick, an' a'thing, what'll I
> dee? I say, rub her wi' Vick. Just fit my mother would have said to
> me, ken.(G19)

Many of the grandmothers said, however, that things were different
now, and they could not interfere in the same way that their own
mothers had done:

> I mean, you'll say, Oh, dinna think that I'm interfering, but if I
> wis *you*, sorta thing. But *my* mother would just have said it. She'd
> come straight out. But J. uses her own—she'll phone, and yet at
> the same time she knows what she's going to do herself.(G33)

Indeed, some said that they deliberately tried not to subject their
own daughters to the same sort of experiences that they had had:

> My mother—we lived with her, you see, when the first three were
> born. And she was inclined to try and take over a bit, you know,
> do this and do that. So I always said I would never interfere.(G53)

'Interfering', they suggested, only caused family trouble:

> I dinna interfere. I dinna believe in that. Because T. could just turn
> roun', an' her man [husband] could turn roun' an' say whit's your
> mother interfering wi' us for!(G4)

and even if they believed in their right to give advice to their own daughter, daughters-in-law (if they had a mother of their own available) were out of bounds:

> Daughter-in-laws, no, that's a different story. I wouldna interfere, they'll follow *their* mothers, like.(G14)

Contrary to the health visitors' impression, the majority of grandmothers said that they would not recommend their own remedies, and that their advice was usually confined to encouraging their daughters to consult a doctor:

> I think they're better wi' the doctor, rather than granny's aul' remedies.(G12)
> They come up and say something's wrong. I just say, well, ging to the doctor. Efter all, your man's peyin' the stamp [National Insurance] for it.(G4)
> She would take my advice up to a point, you know. But if she thought I was speaking a lot of rubbish she would tell me! She says, Oh, Mum! But if it was anything to do with the health of the children she would take my advice and go and see the doctor or call him in.(G11)

Some grandmothers, of course, were rueful about the fact that their daughters scorned their remedies and refused their advice:

> The younger generation now, they've no time for older people at all.(G51)
> I told my daughter-in-law to use olive oil, she just wouldn't do that—Oh no, I'd never put anything in his ears.(G1)
> They turn and say, that's old-fashioned now, so I say nothing! M. has an awful habit of telling me I'm old-fashioned. But I says old-fashioned ways is the best.(G56)

and many emphasised their daughters' independence:

> They tend to think you are interfering with them. The youngsters of today—they don't want to take their parents' advices altogether. They try to be far too independent for that.(G30)
> They just say, don't interfere, Mum, we know what to do! They've got their ways, and we've got our ways, they aye seem to know what to do—they take their ain advice. And they're usually right.(G32)

Indeed, several grandmothers gave the impression, like G32, of being surprised at their daughter's capability. They seemed to be more confident and knowledgeable than they themselves had been at that age:

> I think she's mature for her age, she's been through a lot. I think I rely on her as much as she relies on me. I think she's more capable, actually, than I was.(G41)

The young mothers' accounts of the relationship matched these descriptions very closely, even (as noted previously) when mother–daughter pairs are considered. They were apt to say: yes, you learned from your mother, but in the majority of cases this seemed to be a conventional 'approved' response rather than anything they believed very strongly. A minority of mothers said very explicitly that they based their child-rearing practices or their health care on their mother's example:

> You seem to follow your ma's footsteps. You see her daein' it and you think it's right and you should dae it an' a'! (M27, in fact referring to her grandmother, who brought her up)
> I think ideas are handed down from your own mother and father. You thought what they said was stupid at the time but you do it with your own family.(M24)

The majority of mothers, however, gave the same account of independence and dislike of 'interference' that the grandmother gave. Many agreed that they had relied upon their mothers when their first child had been a baby; a high proportion of our sample was, of course, very young and living with their mothers at that time. Others said that they had never paid very much attention:

> When he was a baby—do this, do that. I just ignored her. I just went my own way.(M35)
> When A. was little it would be, don't do this, and do that, but I just said, Look here, who's bringing up this kid! And she soon stopped. We have different opinions on bringing up kids.(M5)
> I think she's got the message that I'll do things my way.(M41)

Very few said that they believed in their mothers' remedies: 'Your mother often gives you old wives' tales' (M3) and most claimed to prefer up-to-date information from clinics or doctors:

> You go along to the clinic and they tell you exactly what you should be daein'. They dinna gie ye a' these aul' wives' tales.(M12)

For the most part, however, the young women substantiated what their mother had said about her efforts not to interfere, and showed some sympathy and understanding for the grandmother's position:

> No, my mother never gives advice [Husband intervenes to say 'That's a lie, she never stops!'] Well, she'll say, I wouldn't say that. But she won't say, don't. She wouldn't say, you've got to do it, because that would be interfering.(M24)
> My mother had seven kids—she's bound to know something about it . . . but she's never been interfering, or say, dae this and dae that, she'll maybe say, do you think you should?(M12)
> My mother used to try all the home remedies—she did her best

with so many of us. But I think children are healthier nowadays anyway. My mother did her best in the circumstances. She'll give me ideas, but none of them ever worked.(M7)

Familial Patterns in Health-Related Behaviour

It was noted in chapter 11 that the younger generation, as a group, were similar to their mothers in that their early childbearing history had tended to be disturbed, with high rates of youthful, illegitimate and prenuptial pregnancies. Very few of the young mothers appeared likely to bear the large families typical of the previous generation, however: in comparing the family-planning behaviour of mothers and daughters, very different situations are being compared. There were, indeed, one or two families in which both generations had appeared to exhibit some lack of control over contraception, but much more common were grandmothers who described unplanned families, and daughters who had no intention of following their example:

> It wis jist accidents. We didn't have the contraceptions you have nowadays.(G41)
> I'm going to try for another baby when S. is two. I think it's soon enough. You don't have time to give them the proper attention otherwise. My mother said she had hers too quickly.(M41)

Nevertheless, when family sizes were compared in the two generations, there did appear to be some association between larger than average (for the group) families in the two generations (see Table 15.2). There is, however, no evidence that this was due to any

Table 15.2 Family size in mother–daughter pairs[a]

Number of children born to mother (to date):	Number of children born to grandmother	
	1, 2 or 3	4 or more
1 or 2	18 families	7 families
3 or more	8 families	17 families

Note: [a] 50 families on whom there is complete information for the grandmother

continuity of apathetic attitudes, still less to any influence exerted by the older generation. Discussion with both generations tended to dwell upon the desirability and feasibility of limiting fertility nowadays. To a limited extent, it may have been due to teenage pregnancies in some of the higher-parity women of the younger generation, who thus might have been repeating the behaviour of their mothers. In several other cases, however, a larger than average family had been deliberate and planned. The limited data of this small sample cannot be more than suggestive, but it seems possible that a positive wish to have more children than average may be associated with having been a member of a large family. The definition of a 'large' family is now, however, very different.

For other aspects of health-related behaviour in relation to children the comparison between mothers and daughters is not very meaningful, since the norms of behaviour had changed completely. Most grandmothers had at least attempted to breast-feed, for instance, but very few mothers. It can be noted, however, that all the nine young women who had any experience of breast-feeding had mothers who had attempted to breast-feed also.

For the most part the grandmothers said that they had not discussed the question with their daughters:

> She just automatically decided she was going to breast-feed. I'm doing it, she says. I says well, good luck to you.(G37)

One or two of the young mothers said that perhaps they did 'get the idea' from their own mothers, but most grandmothers said simply that it was up to their daughters to decide; they would not interfere. On the other hand, many described their *own* mothers as much more forceful and influential:

> The health visitor *made* me! I tried for two month, I really went through it. I thought, was I feeding her right? And my mother said, in the state I wis putten' mysel' in I wis putten' it onto B., really, so she says to the nurse, she's definitely not able to breast-feed, she says, the baby should go onto the bottle.(G65)

As described in chapter 12, more mothers and daughters spoke of direct advice and influence with regard to infant diets at weaning. Almost all mother–daughter pairs had behaved similarly, according to the grandmothers' accounts and the data from 1950–53, but the behaviour was more strongly disapproved of now than it had been at the time when the young mothers were born.

For other aspects of infant care, such as clinic attendance, there is evidence that the older generation's recollection or presentation may have been very unreliable, and the mother–daughter comparison can be made with confidence only for that half of the sample for which 1950–53 data are available. Of course, the available services have changed, so that like is not being compared with like. Depending on where they were living, clinic attendance was less easy for some of the older generation, and health-visiting services may not have been as well developed. Reliance on old (and not always entirely complete) records may be untrustworthy. However, a judgement can be made that of the 30 grandmothers from the 1950–53 study, there were 10 who were consistently reported as non-attenders at clinics, as missing assessments and special clinic appointments, and as having neglected immunisation for their children. Among their 30 daughters, a much smaller proportion—perhaps 4 women—came into this category. All had in fact had mothers who behaved similarly. On the other hand, it can be noted that 6 of the 'neglectful' among the older generation had daughters whose behaviour was not the same. There is no evidence that, even in the four families where patterns of behaviour seemed to be repeated, attitudes were being 'transmitted' or grandmothers were being actively influential.

Child Care during the Survey Period

The behaviour which was recorded during the six-months' survey period matched very well with the account that both generations had given of their 'usual' actions. The young women were very likely to telephone their mothers or go to see them, but gave the impression of simply wanting to talk rather than seek advice. This was, naturally, most likely if the husband worked away from home. The advice they were given was most usually to consult a doctor, as the grandmothers had said:

I asked my mum but she wasn't willing to give any advice, with D. being a premature baby. She said I should do what the doctors and hospital said.(M6)

Indeed, the young women often said that their mothers 'fussed', and were too anxious to call a doctor. The account of one was:

If I don't know what to do I just phone my mother and she tells me. Mind you, she's a bittie over-protective, the least little thing, she says, you'd better go to the doctor.(M65)

and this was borne out on several occasions during the survey when the same mother reported, about particular symptoms:

I phoned my mother and she said, you'd better get the doctor, just to be on the safe side!(M65)

The 'over-protectiveness' of which the grandmothers were accused was perhaps no more than a very normal reaction to the grandmother role: as one explained:

I worry maybe more about the grandchildren. I mean, I wis aye worried about my own, but you've time to *see* their things and what's going on, whereas wi' your own you're too busy.(G25)

This protectiveness was certainly not displayed in independent action regarding the grandchildren, even though many grandmothers often had the care of them during the day, while the mother was working or out shopping, or as babysitter in the evening. It was notable that the grandmothers always thought it necessary to ask the mother's *permission* before calling a doctor to a sick child. G32, for instance, telephoned her daughter at work to ask if she could send for the doctor for a child who was obviously ill. When a grandchild seemed very ill at G23's house, she was sent home wrapped in blankets in a son's lorry, with the recommendation that a doctor should be called. We have only one instance, among all the 'illness episodes' reported, of a grandmother taking action on her own initiative: G13 took a child to the dentist, when her teeth were still hanging loose two weeks after they had been knocked in an accident.

With regard to child care generally, it was common for the older generation to offer conventional criticisms: the grandchildren stayed up too late, were too indulged, ate too many sweets, were not wrapped up enough against the cold. While mothers complained of the grandparents 'spoiling' the children, the older generation in turn sometimes found them ill-behaved; *their* child-rearing, they said, had been stricter:

> They get awa' wi' things that I wid niver ha' let my ain family get awa' wi'(G6)

On the other hand, the older women might recognise that it was their own stamina that was getting less:

> Many a day I'll say, Oh, me, have I a' this gang the day? But mind you, I wouldnae be pleased if they didna' come!(G1)

and they realised that, as many said, 'times are changed':

> We fussed too much then . . . we were too strict, I think, you know. We held them down too much, ken, when we were bringing them up.(G24)

The overall impression, in the majority of families, is of very loving grandparents who spoke of the children at length, and who often helped their daughters with emotional support and in practical ways. There was, however, very little overt influence on health care or child-rearing practices.

Attitudes to Health and Health Services in Mother–Daughter Pairs
It has been noted that some of the young mothers did think that their own upbringing had influenced them, and believed that they were copying their mothers in a general way. There were, however, few

attitudes that could be identified as deriving directly from the older generation.

Very rarely, a daughter repeated a phrase about health and illness, or about a specific disease, which was recognisable as a favourite of her mother's. (The opposite direction of influence must be considered too, of course, but most conventional wisdoms appeared to derive from the generation with the longer experience and the greater store of anecdote). There were one or two mother/daughter pairs who expressed similar ideas, in particular, about 'family failings' and the place of heredity as a causal factor in disease. On the other hand, there were more who expressed dissimilar ideas. There were mothers who felt pessimistic about the inevitability of ill health, and their daughters who reacted by saying 'I've nae time for folk that's nae weel. My mother's aye got something wrang wi' her, and that annoys me.' There were one or two families in which both mother and daughter expressed the same trust in doctors and liking for a family doctor relationship (perhaps in fact sharing the same doctor), but there were more in which attitudes to health services were very different.

In summary, no consistent relationship could be found between the attitudes of mothers and daughters, despite the close relationship characteristic of the sample. It appeared that inter-generational changes—inextricably bound up with changes in life-style and circumstances, changes in the provision of services, and general changes in public attitudes—were more important than direct familial transmission. The service implications of these conclusions will be discussed in the final chapter.

References

[1] e.g. Sussman, M. B. (1959), 'The isolated nuclear family: fact or fiction', *Social Problems*, **6**, 333.
Sussman, M. B. (1962), 'Parental aid and married children', *Marriage and Family Living*, **24**, 230.
Sweetser, D. A. (1964), Mother–daughter ties between generations in industrial societies, *Family Processes*, **3**, 332.

[2] Litman, T. J. (1971), 'Health care and the family: a three-generational analysis', *Medical Care*, **9**, 67.

16 Conclusions and Service Implications

In this study, we were examining the suggestion that one important reason for poorer health in the children of lower class families was the behaviour, particularly the service-use behaviour, of the mothers (although of course there was no suggestion that this was the only cause: in such a complex area as health, cause can never be single). These behaviours, it was suggested, might be associated with certain attitudes towards health, and these attitudes associated in turn with the attitudes of an older generation. Thus direct familial transmission of attitudes and values could result in poor health care through generations.

An alternative model for the persistence of certain attitudes in socially disadvantaged groups might, it was noted, involve continuity in the environment rather than direct familial transmission. The 'culture of poverty' model often used in the literature on health and health-service use, particularly in the United States, suggests that although of course the social environment changes, and poverty may be differently defined, nevertheless relative poverty remains. Similarly, although health care progresses, it may be that the poor still find structures of service difficult to use or inappropriate for their needs.

Using, in our study, a sample of families selected to provide a stringent test of these hypotheses, neither was supported in the original simple form.

We believe that we have shown that some of the children could indeed be called 'health deprived', and that this deprivation was in part directly associated with the behaviour of the young mothers—that is, it was not, for instance, wholly due to a deficit at birth which could be explained by genetic factors. (And, of course, some of the undoubted deficit which did occur in some children at birth was associated with very youthful childbearing and other behavioural factors.) However, there were also ways in which a disadvantaged environment could be *directly* indicted, with the mothers' behaviour of less importance, and ways, too, in which the services available might themselves be indicted. Accidents are perhaps an example of the first, and poor dental services a partial illustration of the second.

The influence upon the mothers' behaviour of continuity and change in the social environment and in the structure of services, both directly and through their effect upon attitudes, must also not be underestimated. Both have been illustrated in many ways. The circumstances of the women's daily lives inevitably affect the way they perceive their children's symptoms, their service-use behaviour, and their attitudes to health.

There were minor ways in which a 'family health culture' could be demonstrated, and its direct transmission from grandmother to mother, as well as a persisting set of subcultural beliefs. Ideas about infant feeding might be instanced here, or fear of chest complaints, or (at a more general level) a sturdy belief that 'lying down to illness' was a moral weakness.

On the other hand, many mother–daughter pairs were quite different in their attitudes, and their social or geographical closeness was not associated with the variation. Mothers and daughters who saw each other every day might express quite differing views. Whether the analysis is of beliefs and values in general, or of the actual action taken during the survey period and the reasons given for that action, the *direct* familial link appeared to be weak.

Viewed as groups rather than individual pairs, the attitudes of the two generations to curative service-use were conspicuously different. For the majority of grandmothers, low expectations of present-day services (which they saw as a deterioration from the 'family doctor' service which was their ideal) were associated with low reported service use. This group of middle-aged women is, of course, one which is often accused of 'over-use' of primary care, and we have little evidence of the relationship between the grandmothers' accounts and their actual behaviour. It was clear, however, that many of their conditions had been neglected in the past and their norms of health were low. At the present time their tolerance for pain and discomfort was high, and they were not conspicuously among those who are said to be queuing up at their practitioners' surgeries for psychotropic drugs or the alleviation of menopausal syndromes.

On the other hand, most of the younger generation, although their concept of 'normal health' continued to be low, had high expectations of curative medicine. They saw many services as a 'right' and expected a great deal of medication for their children. Few retained the deferential model characteristic of their mothers: they had adopted new attitudes to meet new circumstances, though in some cases, because of their lack of skills in dealing with a more complex system than their mothers had known, these attitudes might lead to troubled service-use.

Where the environment had changed least—that is, where the young mothers were in the most disadvantaged circumstances—one set of attitudes had remained unchanged. This group was characterised, as their mothers had been, by a disorganised and sometimes apathetic approach to preventive care.

Thus the model which represents our conclusion is complex: we found a degree of continuity, but attitudes were related to behaviour sometimes in the same way in the two generations, and sometimes differently. The children cannot all be called generally 'health deprived'. Nevertheless, in certain circumstances and in particular ways, deprivation does persist.

Service Implications

Throughout, we have made suggestions about the ways in which medical practices or patterns of service-delivery were found to be ineffective in safeguarding the health of these children. We would not suggest that total solutions are easy or even possible, since the environmental factors remain. However, we summarise here some of the service factors which seemed to us to be important. Since structures of service will differ from place to place, some of these may be particular to the area of the study. The problems observed are certainly not due, however, to a general poverty of services in the City where the women lived. The area had the advantage, for the purpose of the research, of favourable characteristics (except perhaps for dentistry) by all the conventional measures of service-provision. Its citizens commonly express pride in its health services, and several of our respondents echoed this traditional view. An attempt will of course be made in the suggestions which follow to focus more upon general principles than upon local systems.

First, we would distinguish those 'inefficiencies' in the use of medical services (by which we mean both overuse and underuse, conflict or worry generally, and 'excess' as well as inadequacy of service-supply) which we suggest are inevitable, from those 'inefficiencies' which could be remedied. We would suggest that perhaps the conflicts and dissatisfactions described by some women in each generation are (in different ways) an inevitable response to a changing health service. Compared with the (perhaps idealised) form of service favoured by the older generation, the structure of services has become more differentiated, bureaucratic and businesslike: one must telephone for appointments, one may not know the doctor who comes, the onus is more upon the patient (they feel) to know what his needs are. The older women bewail the passing of the service they were used to, and a younger generation adapts to the service they experience now.

The confusion expressed by our respondents about their expectations of doctors, particularly in primary care, is perhaps no more than a reflection of some uncertainty about their proper function among the doctors themselves. Just as there may be some tension between, at one extreme, the idea of family practice as an all-embracing service in which personal guidance is emphasised and preventive medicine has a place, and at the other a model of primary care which leaves more responsibility to the patient, simply responding efficiently to demand, so there may be matching tensions in the expectations of the patients.

We would also suggest that it is inevitable that the mothers of very young children (in every social class, though perhaps to the greatest extent where the mothers are most burdened) will be inefficient users of medical services, and 'difficult' from the providers' point of view. The mothers of babies are always going to be apt to call doctors to the house in the middle of the night for respiratory infections; the mothers of handicapped children are always going to be anxious, and seek for more information than it is possible to give. These things are inherent in the situation of having children to care for. That some conflict and seemingly irrational behaviour is inevitable is all the more reason, however, for tackling inefficiencies which could be solved.

At the first and most fundamental level of *primary care*, we would suggest that the potential effectiveness of generalised health education in curbing what is seen as overuse of service for trivialities is severely limited. Specific education by doctors was, however, something which the mothers expressed appreciation of and need for. Many demonstrated considerable worry because they did not know, in many circumstances, whether professional advice and treatment was appropriate or not; those who *had* been told exactly what signs and symptoms to look out for, in a particular child, were notably more decisive in their actions. Others might worry over symptoms for hours or days, only to find them disappearing as the doctor arrived; ruefully, they acknowledged that their behaviour might seem irrational and in the event over-anxious. In fairness, it must be added that a large proportion of these women's GPs appeared to understand the problems of knowing when a small child was ill, and appreciate the occasional inevitable 'panicking' of mothers, and they gave very willing and uncomplaining service. It was noted, however, that quite frequently mothers might reach the stage where they would be reluctant to seek help—and this time it might be serious—because they were quite sure that 'the doctor must be sick of me'.

What the mothers would most have appreciated would have been 'education' in the form of a set of simple rules applicable to *this* child, with information about what was serious and what was not. As was noted, very few even owned a thermometer and among those who did there were very varied views on what degree of fever signalled danger. Also, the few doctors who were willing to speak to mothers on the telephone probably saved themselves many unnecessary journeys. The possibility of giving telephoned advice is, of course, a problematic area: some practitioners might see it as a very imperfect form of doctoring, and others might fear the opening of floodgates to an endless stream of inquiries. It has to be added that there were a few occasions on which mothers expressed dissatisfaction at 'doctors diagnosing over the telephone'. We would suggest that the women's high expectations of the service—their belief that they had a right to an immediate visit from the doctor if they thought it justified—were crucial in these cases. Nevertheless, though it is not within our competence to judge the precise number of occasions, it is certain that many of the rather high level of housecalls demanded by our families could have been replaced—to the mother's complete satisfaction—by a minute's conversation.

On the other hand, when the mothers clearly saw an emergency, their urgent worry was that the doctor should come *at once*: indeed, few had cause for serious complaint. Inefficiency on both sides—'unnecessary' calls or delay in responding to calls—seemed alike to arise because there was no middle way for the mothers to choose. Either the child had to be fit to be taken out, or fit to wait (perhaps several days) until a surgery appointment could be obtained, or else the doctor had to be brought to the house.

He might come more willingly, of course, if it did not mean travelling to the other side of the city. One of the ways in which our data surprised us was to find, as reported in chapter 14, how many of our families were registered with doctors a considerable distance from their homes, and how common it was for different members of the family to be registered with different practices. (It has to be remembered that 'distance' might be measured differently for the doctor, travelling by car, and the patient, dependent on bus services; it might well be easier to travel by bus to the centre of town from an outlying housing estate than to reach a geographically nearer crosscity practice.) It may be argued that the enforced rationalisation of practices would be strongly resisted by patients as an infringement of their right to a choice of doctor. As we have noted, however, the majority of the young mothers did not feel very strongly about a personal relationship with their general practitioner. Many would have changed if it had been made easy for them to do so (the daunting nature of the present procedures to people like our respondents is not perhaps appreciated by administrators) and if they had still been able to choose from among a group—especially if they could choose different doctors for different purposes. As the number of health centres and large group practices increases, this possibility becomes more likely.

We indicated clearly in chapter 9 that we believed our mothers' problems in the area of *dental care* were not altogether of their own making. A true 'cycle of deprivation' was in operation here: because many mothers had no long-standing relationship with a dentist of their own, they found it very difficult to obtain even emergency treatment, and because it was so difficult to find treatment, problems worsened or were neglected. Then, when the treatment was eventually obtained, it was necessarily drastic and unpleasant, and the families were seen as 'bad' and neglectful patients.

Some mothers used the school dental services happily, but for those who would not or could not (because children were not allowed out of school alone to attend, no matter how near by, and the timing might not be convenient for working mothers) repeated examinations at school with no way of ensuring that treatment followed appeared to be a waste of time.

Health education has obviously had little effect on the traditionally poor dental health of this social and geographical group, and it is clear from many of the quotations in chapter 9 that their definition of dental problems as natural, inevitable and irrelevant to health should be countered by the provision of information. The popularity among a few mothers in our sample of group dental practices based in two local health centres may point the way to making treatment and preventive care more accessible and acceptable. Meanwhile, it would be profitable if health visitors could become as involved in dental care as they are in other aspects of child health and development, since there were in our sample many children below school age (often as young as two and three) who were suffering considerable pain unnecessarily.

It is clear that the *health-visiting service* was an important source of help and support to many of our mothers, especially at the time when their first child was young. A few problems arose, as we have indicated in various chapters: the area concerned is better serviced with health-visiting services than many others, but staff shortages in the past and movement of staff had sometimes led to families being under-visited or subjected to many changes of health visitor; there were particular conflicts over infant feeding; the ways in which the children might obtain immunisation sometimes presented health visitors with difficulties in ensuring that records were up to date; and the feeling of some mothers that they were always potentially under suspicion of 'non-accidental injury' or neglect sometimes damaged their relationship with health visitors and with clinics. Obviously, from the client's point of view continuity of health-visiting personnel is very important: this has, however, to be reconciled with the needs of training or the possible desire of health visitors for change and varied experience. Continuity is, however, particularly necessary in the poorer areas where social problems may be greatest and the need for energetic follow-up (of, for instance, chronic conditions or non-immunisation) essential. It was suggested to us by some health visitors that these were in fact areas where movement of staff was, for various reasons, likely to be most frequent.

Our mothers were apt to favour the attachment of health visitors to general practices or health centres, which is of course increasingly common. This enabled them, in some cases, to see the health visitor and the service as part of an integrated *health* service, rather than as simply visits from someone they could rarely name, whose function they were unsure of.

Difficulties obviously remain in the relationship between some doctors and health visitors. Particularly where health visitors were not attached to practices (but sometimes even if they were) we noted that their information about medical events was not always as full as it might usefully have been. No health visitor talked to us about problems in their relationship with doctors, but it was obvious that occasionally their position was extremely difficult. They might be torn between their traditional relationship, as nurses, with the medical profession, and their identification with distressed or complaining clients. Their role might formally be seen as relating only to child care or preventive medicine, but inevitably they would be involved in the child's—or even the parent's—illnesses. Some families also chose to use them very much as social workers. In general, it would seem that their role, which is undoubtedly a crucial one, requires clarification.

One minor point perhaps worthy of mention is that there was not, among our families, any reaction against male health visitors, nor did those whom we interviewed suggest that they experienced any problems in gaining acceptance.

Despite our mothers' majority opinion that *child health clinics* were greatly valued for young babies, some confusion did arise between the functions of clinic doctor and GP. It may be, of course, that these women were using the clinics (for older children) in a way which was not intended; the convenience of siting and openness or difficulty of access of practices is again relevant. The mothers believed, however, that the clinic doctors could diagnose but could not prescribe, and they found this difficult to understand. Obviously, they preferred clinics where they might see their own GP.

Our families' very free use of the *accident and emergency service* of the children's hospital might add fuel to the intermittent controversy which arises about 'inappropriate' use of these facilities. This we would deplore: in fact, as we have noted, our mothers were almost unanimous in their appreciation of what was, to them, an important safety net. Indeed, it could be argued that the use of the accident and emergency service at night, or during weekends, or on occasions when it was thought that X-rays might be required, or when only a simple examination or dressing was necessary, was a more efficient use of professional time than trying to contact a general practitioner. The patient came to the service rather than vice versa, nurses were available to provide minor dressings, and if the condition were only trivial a minimum of professional time was wasted. From the mothers' point of view, they were happy to know that they did not have to ask for service, or make out a case to receptionists whom they thought unsympathetic: the service was there, and always (in their experience) willingly provided. If it did, after all, appear to be unnecessary fussing on their part, at least they had caused minimum trouble. One family not formally included in the sample, because the series of visits was not completed, was of 'tinker' origin and always spent the summer travelling. This mother had admitted very freely that she *never* used a general practitioner, but always expected accident and emergency departments of hospitals to provide primary care; she was extremely happy with the service she received.

Our mothers were all fortunate enough, of course, to be within relatively easy reach of an accident and emergency department. We would suggest not that the use of such departments should be made more restrictive, but rather that the principle might profitably be applied in large health centres, group practices, and medical depart ments of children's hospitals.

In connection with *specialist services*, the major problem was the perception of these women that the system was fragmented and the lines of responsibility unclear. The information they were given (or, more usually, the lack of it) suggested to them that communication between hospital specialists, general practitioner, clinic doctors, and school health services, was sometimes lacking. They also felt that they, the parents, with their very particular knowledge of their child, were not accepted as members of the team. It also seemed to them that problems of management and behaviour—learning difficulties, enuresis, behaviour problems, speech difficulties—were separated out, and assigned to social workers, health visitors, or specialist therapists. To the mothers, however, it was usually clear that these were only part of medical problems, and should be considered in that context.

The questions of the identification of *handicap* and the expressed desire of mothers for more information about diagnosis and prognosis (where our study's findings have frequently been suggested before) is, of course, a very difficult one. One point which we would wish to make, however, is that in discussion of this problem it often appears to be assumed that 'the giving of information' is one discrete act, performed by a specialist on one occasion or deliberately controlled over a few interactions. But of course, as our data show, parents obtain their information from a multitude of sources which cannot be controlled—from the media, from their mothers, from the subcultural stock of 'knowledge', from their own and their family's experience, from general practitioners, health visitors and other health professionals, from the surreptitious reading of records and from the symbolic meanings they assign (rightly or wrongly) to procedures. For instance, more than one mother mentioned to us the significance of the exact placing of the baby's cot in the Special Nursery. Professional discussions of 'how is it best to tell parents?' or 'How much do parents understand of what they are told, in particular ways and at particular times?' often forget to ask the essential initial question: 'What knowledge, right or wrong, do they already have of this situation or this condition?'

We noted that the designation of children as '*At Risk*', especially on the grounds of adverse birth conditions, had been reasonably efficient, in this sample, in selecting out those children likely to suffer poorer health some years after birth. We have to add, however, that we could find no evidence that the identification or treatment of handicaps (sight, hearing, convulsions, speech and behaviour problems) had been more readily achieved in the children known to be 'At Risk'. We can have no knowledge, of course, of what would have happened had these children *not* been subject to special monitoring. But the mothers' accounts of their interactions with their general practitioners do not always suggest, for instance, that the doctor was specially alert to the possibility of handicap in these cases.

Some Research Implications

Finally, we must note that of course this is only one small, intensive and local study. The generalisability of our findings remains to be tested in many ways. We cannot know whether the same mechanisms explain the persistence of health disadvantage in social groups of other kinds or in other places, nor whether the relationship between attitudes and behaviour over the generations is the same in more fortunate social circumstances. Since we have emphasised the importance of the structure of health services in its effect upon both attitudes and behaviour, the particular nature of local structures, both past and present, must be an important variable.

There are many questions we should like to ask. Is the absence of a positive concept of health one of the special marks of social disadvantage, as we have suggested? Is the 'accelerated' nature of these women's lives, with early childbearing, grandmotherhood, and resignation to being 'past it' in their 20s and 'getting on now' in their 40s, similarly a special feature of the lives of disadvantaged women? How would the interpretation of children's symptoms differ in a better-educated group of young mothers? Many of our young mothers' lives were difficult, but they were, as a group, very home-centred, working (if at all) because they needed money: it was not a group in which we were likely to find career-women, or those who had very salient areas of life beyond their husbands, children, and extended families. How would the principles of service-use differ in such a group? We noted that the young mothers were in general quite high users of curative services, but that *within* our sample it was those who were in the better social and environmental circumstances who were more likely to make most use of services. This would suggest that high expectations of medicine are likely to accompany increasing prosperity, but we do not know at what point (if at all) increasing education might begin to curb dependence on medical services. We were, deliberately, examining a group who were neither upwardly nor downwardly socially mobile, up to the present time. Groups of considerable interest would be those who are now in the same social circumstances as our families, but have brought with them a different background and family history, and those who share the background of our families but have escaped to a different life-style.

We did not (in the interests of limiting our data to manageable proportions) seek to examine closely both sides of the doctor–patient interaction, but focused upon the patients' perspectives. Of course, completeness requires more direct study of how the *doctors* viewed these symptoms and these demands upon their services.

We were not able, either, to consider adequately the *husband's* role in health care, or to look at male/female differences in either attitudes or consulting behaviour. There is no doubt that we were right to anticipate that it would be the women of the families who would be eager to talk about health matters, and similar interviews with an older generation of men would probably have been much more difficult. We are left, however, without any knowledge of whether the disadvantaged (and in occupational terms often more physically taxing) lives of men had been associated with similar attitudes to health. These are only some of the further questions raised by this study.

At a more general level, our intensive acquaintance with this small group of families has, we believe, shown particularly how badly more sophisticated and more up to date categorisations of social disadvantage and social class are needed. By the conventional social groupings of the Registrar General, the families studied were all categorised as social class IV or V. At the particular stage of the life-cycle exemplified by our young families, however, we have noted that there was a great deal of rapid and sometimes erratic change—from unemployment to employment, from one sort of job to another, and from extreme poverty to relative affluence. In any case, no social class is homogeneous, and diversity is likely particularly at the top or bottom of the scale. Nor is any particular class likely to have exactly the same characteristics in urban and rural settings, in different geographical areas, and over periods of time. Our group of families did, to a considerable extent, exhibit the features of subculture, but it was one based on geography, social history, and economic circumstances rather than on simply belonging to the class of wage-earners in semi-skilled or unskilled jobs.

Although the 'social classes' which have been used for such a long period of time for large-scale statistics have the advantage of continuity, the crude' division by occupation may be becoming increasingly unreal. For practical purposes, attempts to refine the concept of social class (such as the Hope–Goldthorpe scale),[1] or to produce indices of social disadvantage (such as the Social Index of the research programme *Child Health and Education in the Seventies*),[2] may be more profitable.

Conclusion

Above all, we suggest that our data have shown the inadequacy of simple models of 'illness behaviour', and the dangers of applying what may well be out-of-date concepts to changing societies. In many ways, the grandmother generation did fit the model summarised as the 'culture of poverty'. They did not appear to be efficient or demanding users of services, and their attitudes could be said to be characterised by apathy, a feeling of powerlessness, and low norms of health. The psychological characteristics which have been said to accompany these attitudes, in the classic studies of the 'culture of poverty' model applied to health-care behaviour were not, however, conspicuous: we found little evidence in this lively group of 'a lack of identity, low self-evaluation, and a weak perception of self'.[3] Nor were they 'more likely to accept the role of the sick' or 'have a high regard for self as sick'.[4]

In a sense, their values were *more* consonant with those of service-providers than were the values of their daughters, who were even less recognisable as fitting the 'culture of poverty' model. It seems possible that the ideal model of the general practitioner, for instance, as it is still presented in the media or in fiction, and perhaps still presented by the profession themselves, is more akin to the grandmothers' model than the mothers'. The older women's expectations of the doctor—as a family friend who is at the same time the unquestioned expert—are higher than those of the younger women, but their demands on him are less. It may be that they presented themselves as having less overt conflict with their doctors because this is the model which the doctors themselves find attractive.

The younger generation were found to be more varied. Some had retained this model, but combined it with higher expectations in terms of the actual items of service supplied. Others had rejected the older model, adopting values and behaviour which fitted better to the pattern of services which was more likely actually to exist. Still others among the mothers had fallen between stools—they had rejected the 'family friend' model of the doctor, but found themselves dealing with a complex pattern of services which put them in some ways at even more of a disadvantage. Service initiatives based on the paternalistic model appropriate to their mothers were not always acceptable; on the other hand, a 'consumerist' model implies, if it is to be equitable, an ability to make use of what is available. The young women still lacked the skills, education, and stable social environment which would have made dealing with the system easy. Changed attitudes had led to changed behaviour in many ways, but the result—troubled service-use—was often the same.

References

[1] Goldthorpe, J. H. and Hope, K. (1974), *The Social Grading of Occupations*, Oxford: Clarendon Press.

[2] Osborn, A. F. and Morris, T. C. (1978), *The Rationale for a Composite Index of Social Class and its Evaluation*, Mimeo, University of Bristol.

[3] Rainwater, L. (1968), 'The lower class: health, illness and medical institutions' in Deutscher, I. and Thompson, E. J. (eds.), *Among the People: Encounters with the Poor*, New York: Basic Books.

[4] Rosengren, W. R. (1964), 'Social class and becoming ill' in Shostak, A. and Gomberg, W. (eds.) *Blue Collar World*, Englewood Cliffs, N.J.: Prentice-Hall.

Appendix A A Note on the Selection of the Families

In the original 1950–53 sample of Thompson and Illsley there were 455 women, of all social classes. It was thought of interest to include as many as possible of these women's families, although it had not been expected that many would be available, after more than 25 years, who filled the rather complicated criteria for inclusion: grandmother in social class IV or V at the time of her delivery, grandmother still alive and still living in the City, grandmother having had a daughter, her daughter having had children herself in the same City, being in social class IV or V at the time, and still living in the City. A total of 124 young families were identified from the maternity records as being potentially likely to fill the criteria. Of these, 90 were found not in fact to do so, since the older woman was dead, either generation had moved away from the City, or the family was simply not now traceable. To add to the potential sample, 87 young families were identified from the maternity records, with a mother who was born in the City, and in which the grandmother would at least be of the same generation as the 1950–53 sample though not in fact a subject of that study. In a similar way, 51 of these were untraceable or found not to fill the criteria.

After a small pilot study, letters were written to all the young mothers potentially thought to be suitable, asking them if their mother was living in the City, and if so whether they would be willing to take part in the study. Of the 70 who were in fact eligible, 4 replied by letter declining, and 23 replied by letter agreeing. Personal visits were made to the remainder (and, of course, to many more who had not replied but who were found not to fill the criteria). Of the 43 eligible families who had not replied, 6 declined when visited and 37 agreed. The point may be made that, in this particular social group, reliance on postal replies is likely to be unprofitable, and non-reply certainly does not mean that the respondents are reluctant to take part in research.

We could not be sure, when initially accepting the young family into the series, that the grandmother would be equally willing to participate, and there are in fact 47 interviews with the older generation. In a few cases the grandmother eventually declined to be interviewed, one died and one moved away, and there are two pairs of sisters among the young mothers. In three cases, the 'grandmother' is in fact the young mother's mother-in-law; where her own mother was dead and the paternal grandmother was close by and seen frequently, it seemed acceptable to include her in the place of the maternal grandmother. The relationship in these cases seemed very similar to that in the other families: the mother-in-law had adopted completely the role typical of the maternal grandmothers.

It must be stressed that a great deal was being asked of the families, over an extended period, and their willingness to co-operate was remarkable. None of the 60 families originally included in the series terminated their participation during the survey period, though the disturbed lives of a few did present some practical difficulties in maintaining regular contact. One family was relinquished because of distress over a bereavement, and another moved away, leaving a final series of 58 young families.

The design of the research meant that a truly random sample was hardly possible, though we have no reason to think that these families are not typical of their social group. The series is defined simply as a group of families who have been in this City and these social classes for at least two generations. Those who have dispersed geographically, and those who up to the last child's birth had been upwardly mobile, are by definition excluded. It must be noted that the three-generational design will also be likely to exclude those families who are most unstable.

Appendix B The Index of 'Disadvantage'

In order to examine the association of social circumstances with possible differences in attitudes and behaviour within the sample, it was necessary to categorise families on some dimension of relative disadvantage. It must be noted that of course none could be called advantaged: none was wealthy, most had received a minimum amount of education, and all had been categorised occupationally as semi- or unskilled working class families in the maternity records from which the series was derived. Initially it had been thought that the categorisation might be easily if crudely made by distinguishing 'good' from 'bad' housing areas.

In fact, this simple design proved to be inadequate, and a multi-dimensional score of relative disadvantage was developed. By coincidence, 29 of the families were scored as 'more' disadvantaged, and 29 as 'less'. The categorisation is not, we would emphasise, presented as an absolute or universally applicable one: it is relative within this group of families, and intended to cover those dimensions of social circumstances which might be expected to have a potential *effect* upon health behaviour.

It may be useful to summarise some of the problems which were met. Firstly, it was obvious that three dimensions had to be separated, and any one of them would have been meaningless on its own. The economic circumstances of the family had to be considered separately from the environmental, and the social circumstances from both. The wages which the family earned were not necessarily correlated with the standard of housing they occupied, and within the household families earning the same amount might choose to spend it in very different ways, providing different environments for the children. In the worst environments one would, as might be expected, find some socially troubled families with disturbed marital relationships: on the other hand, several single-handed mothers with the most conflict-full marital histories had been allocated relatively good housing in the better environments.

Within each of these three dimensions there were also problems and anomalies. In considering the disadvantage suffered by the *children*, is the relevant income measure an absolute one of pounds per week, or the objective problems (debts, inability to buy essential items) of the mother, or the subjective perception of the mother that she does have problems? All these may, of course, be different. Because of this, and also because although we inquired into each family's finances we have no proof, in most cases, about the accuracy of what they said, we decided that the mother's expression of money worries must bear some weight, but not be accepted by itself as an indicator of economic disadvantage: the only objective categorisation was to select out those families definitely at the lowest end of the income scale who were eligible for Family Income Supplement (FIS) or living on social-security payments. Even this, however, might not always be decisive, for during the six-months' survey circumstances could change rapidly, and a short period on social security might not present great hardship to a family with allowances for several children.

The 'social' index is not, we think, entirely adequate. The family environment of the child depends very much on the characters, life-styles, child-centredness, emotional stability, and other characteristics of the parents which we were not competent to measure, and which we could not in any case consider independently from the mother's health behaviour. Yet at the extreme, we felt that to be the child of a single-handed mother, or of a family where there was obvious marital conflict, had to be taken into account as a dimension of 'disadvantage'.

For the 'environmental' index we had again to reconcile anomalies. The poorest dwellings were likely to be found in the poorest estates, but this was not necessarily true: there might be a perfectly adequate dwelling on the edge of, but technically within, a poor estate, and one run-down old block of flats might be found surrounded by better dwellings. The inside fittings and equipment of a flat might similarly be anomalous.

Although we were selecting only the 'more' or 'less' disadvantaged relative to our sample, the fact that the 'environmental' component of the index is more salient than the other two, in that a greater proportion of the families were categorised as 'bad', does indicate some use on our part of absolute standards. The families did seem to us to be more likely to be characterised by a poor environment than by extreme poverty or obviously disturbed family relationships.

It may be that the eventual classification of the families into the 'more' and the 'less' disadvantaged represents no more than subjective judgement. The system of scoring eventually used, which is presented below, has however two functions: firstly, it makes the basis of this judgement explicit, and secondly, it was useful as a means of discipline when trying to compare the weight of different sorts of disadvantage, or categorise families who were borderline cases. The items listed are not, of course, an exclusive list of items which *might* be relevant. Others were considered, tried out on the data, and rejected because *in our sample* they did not appear to be useful or to distinguish families clearly. An example might be the extent and coherence of the extended family, where our sample obviously has special characteristics. There were a few families where this coherence was less than we had presumed when accepting them into the sample, but they were too few for the characteristic to be useful analytically. Another example might be the use which we attempted to make of various official assessments, including health visitor yearly assessments of the family, as noted in the child's records. These demonstrated to us only how difficult any objective assessment of 'home conditions' or the mother's 'care' must be, since there were often inconsistencies in different assessments made of the same family. This attempt was therefore abandoned.

Components of Index of 'Disadvantage'

A. Physical environment

0	1	2
Good housing estate	Intermediate housing estate	Notoriously bad housing estate
Flat or house in good repair, set in clean and pleasant surroundings	Intermediate condition of dwelling	Flat or house run down, exterior environment dirty and dangerous
Furnishing, decoration and equipment of home good	Furnishing and equipment only adequate	Lack of certain items of basic equipment in home
Not overcrowded: less than 2 people/bedroom	—	Overcrowded: more than 2 people/bedroom

Score of 0: 'Good'   Score of 1–3: 'Intermediate'   Score of 4+: 'Bad'

B. Economic circumstances

0	1	2
Mother presents no money problems	Mother presents some worries over money during 6 months; or mother working because of expressed need for money	Family living on social security or at FIS level during 6 months
Breadwinner employed all of 6 months	Breadwinner unemployed at some time during 6 months	Breadwinner un-employed for whole of 6 months
—	Breadwinner Registered Disabled	—
Breadwinner not absent from work with illness for more than 3 days at a time during 6 months	Breadwinner absent from work for prolonged period during 6 months	Breadwinner absent from work with ill-ness for whole of 6 months

Score of 0: 'Good'   Score of 1–3: 'Intermediate'   Score of 4+: 'Bad'

C. Marital relationships and social stability

0	1	2
Stable marriage	History of period(s) of separation in the past, though appears stable now	Divorced, separated, or single-handed parent
No criminal history	History of imprisonment of husband in past	Imprisonment of husband during survey
No official suspicion at any time of neglect or child abuse	Suspicion raised at some time of child neglect or abuse by either parent	Evidence of child abuse by either parent
Marital relationship appears to be good	Some conflict in marriage apparent	Evidence of severe conflict, usually of wife-battering
Score of 0: 'Good'	Any scores in column 1 only: 'Intermediate'	Any scores in column 2: 'Bad'

| | Number of families assessed as: | | |
	'Bad'	'Intermediate'	'Good'
A. Physical environment	22	11	25
B. Economic circumstances	11	9	38
C. Social stability	9	8	41

Overall index

'Less disadvantaged': 29 families

Families assessed as 'good' on A, B and C, or 'intermediate' on only one dimension.

'More disadvantaged': 29 families

Families assessed as 'bad' on any dimension, or 'intermediate' on more than one.

Index

family size, 14, 19, 120, 179
finances, 21, 200, 203
health, 23
housing, 20, 91, 202
husbands, 21, 154, 194
infant nutrition, 131
lay referral, 153
lay remedies, 150
occupations, 21
perception of illness, 49–66
relationship with doctors, 64, 79, 160, 187
relationship with mothers, 174–83
use of clinics, 166, 170, 181, 191
use of services, 42, 64, 95, 164, 171, 187, 195

National Child Development Survey, 3, 45, 88, 99, 108
National Health Service, 17, 164
Non-accidental injury, 96, 169
Normalisation, 31, 64
Norms of health, 28, 185
Nursery schools, 25
Nutrition
  child, 136–43
  infant, 128–36

Obesity, 30
Occupations, 16, 21, 22
Older generation sample, see 'Grandmother' generation
Oral contraception, 37, 122
Otitis media, 68, 71
Outpatient clinics, 42, 80
  for accidents, 90

Perinatal conditions, 69
Pharmacists, 154
Polio immunisation, 168
Practice
  distribution, 165
  group, 189
  organisation, 164, 188
'Predisposing' factors, 2
Pregnancy, 31, 37
Prematurity, 69

Prenuptial conception, 19, 70
Preventive care, 2, 29, 171, 181, 186
  dental, 102
  immunisation, 108
Primary care, 45, 159, 187
Prognosis, 35
Proprietary medicines, 145, 151

Rates of
  accident, 88
  adverse birth conditions, 69
  consultation, 43
  chronic illness, 70
  handicap, 68
  hospitalised illness, 90
  illness, 40
  infant morbidity, 71
Receptionists, 167
Register, At Risk, 73, 192
Rejection of illness, 34
Remedies, 145–52, 178

Safety
  environmental, 91
  in the home, 93
Sample, 8, 197
School health service, 171
  dental service, 104, 189
Service-use, 2, 42–8, 64, 76, 95, 164, 171, 187
Services, health, 186–93
  accident and emergency, 95–8, 191
  child health clinics, 43, 46, 166, 169, 180
  dental, 100, 104–107, 189
  general practitioner, 45, 159, 187
  health visiting, 167, 189
  hospital, 80
  primary care, 45, 159, 187
  school health, 171
  specialist, 43, 80, 191
Smoking, 29
Social class, 194
  and consultation rates, 44
  dental care, 99
  immunisation, 107

Special nursery, 69, 81
Specialist services, 43, 80, 191
Squint, 68, 77, 79
Sterilisation, 119, 124
Stigma
  and handicap, 85
  injury, 87
Stomach pain, 55
Subcultural values, 2
Supplementary feeding, 134
Surgery consultations, 43
Susceptibility, 36
Symptoms, 49–65

Teething, 54
Telephone consultations, 45, 188
Tenements, 91
'Toddies', 150
Tooth decay, 99–107
Tower blocks, 91
Triggers, illness, 50
Triple immunisation, 108
Trivial symptoms, 53, 64, 187

Unemployment, 22
Unhappiness and illness, 33
Urinary infections, 56

Vasectomy, 124
Vitamins, 143

'Weaknesses', 58
Weaning, 134, 180
Whooping-cough, 113
World Health Organisation, 26

Younger generation sample, see
  'Mother' generation

Author Index
Aitken-Swan, J., 127
Alberman, E.D., 5, 87
Alpert, J. J., 66
Andersen, R., 6
Anderson, O. W., 6
Antonovsky, A., 5, 6
Apple, D., 65
Askham, J., 118, 127

Banks, M. H., 48
Beal, J. F., 107
Beresford, S. A. A., 48
Berg, O., 38
Blaney, R., 13, 48
Blaxter, M., 5, 39
Blomfield, J. M., 98
Brandon, S., 87
Brotherston, Sir J., 5
Bury, M. R., 35, 39
Butler, N. R., 5, 48, 87, 98, 107,
  117, 144
Butterfield, W. J. H., 13, 48

Campbell, J. D., 66
Cartwright, A., 13, 66, 155
Chamberlain, A., 127
Chapman, S. S., 6
Coburn, D., 6
Colley, J. R. T., 87
Colombo, J. J., 6
Corkhill, R. T., 87
Court, S. D. M., 87, 98

Davie, R., 5, 7, 48, 87, 98, 107,
  117, 144
Davis, M., 5
DiCocco, L., 65
Dickson, S., 107
Douglas, J. W. B., 87, 98, 144
Dunnell, K., 155
Dutton, D., 6

Eisenberg, L., 26, 38
Erde, E. L., 32, 38

Fabrega, H., 4, 7, 26, 38
Field, D., 26, 38
Fox, J., 98
Freeborn, D. K., 6
Freeman, H., 5
Freidson, E., 155

Goldthorpe, J. H., 196
Goldstein, H., 5, 48, 87, 98, 117,
  144, 151
Gordon, G., 66
Gray, L. C., 6
Greenlick, M. R., 6